Weight Loss for Women 40+

2 Books in 1 Power Pack

Simple and Effective Weight Loss Hacks Plus 28-Day Food, Fitness, and Habit Journal | Planner | Tracker

Kate M. Right

Contents

Weight Loss Hacks for Women Over 40

Feel Lighter and More Energetic Starting Week 1

Kate M. Right

Introduction

After women turn 40, we should feel more comfortable in our own skin. We are wiser, more experienced, and better at dealing with new challenges in life. We know who we are and what we want. We know what is more important in life, and many care less about what others think of us.

However, there is one dreadful fact that most women over 40 cannot escape from - weight gain, even if we eat and exercise the same way as we did before turning 40. Extreme dieting or over exercising is painful and not sustainable. Taking diet pills can have some serious side effects on our health. For those who have the financial means to go through fat removal procedures, you are expected to experience varying degrees of discomfort after each procedure, and you can still gain weight after the procedure.

Many women, myself included, at one point, gave ourselves excuses or legitimate reasons for gaining weight, such as giving birth or raising a family while juggling a career, so there is less time to take care of ourselves. And we tried to convince ourselves that our significant others should love us no matter how our bodies change. That might be true to some extent, but it is absolutely irresponsible to our physical and mental health by allowing ourselves to gain excess weight, meaning gaining more than 10 lbs over our normal weight.

I will certainly not BS you by saying it is OK to gain more weight as we age. There is no reason for women over 40 to settle for less. Managing our weight is not just for looking good; it is critical to our physical and mental health. I will spare you the pain of sitting through big scientific analyses. I will not give a pep talk to get you to exercise more in the gym. I will not bore you with generic tips.

This book is intended to share simple, easy, and practical hacks that you can apply on a daily basis, and soon, you will become a master of effectively managing your weight in a natural and sustainable fashion. Applying even a subset of the hacks listed in this book, you will start feeling leaner and more energetic as soon as week one! Let's get started!

Chapter 1: Fundamentals - Understand Barriers

Before we get into the solution space, let's first make sure you truly understand and can identify your barriers to achieving your health and fitness goals.

Health and fitness goals do not just refer to achieving your weight in your 20s or fitting into clothes you wore in your 20s, which can be achieved by applying hacks listed in this book. However, there are other health indicators that you need to monitor to achieve holistic health and fitness goals. Is your BMI (body mass index) in the healthy range? Are your cholesterol and insulin levels in the healthy range? Do you feel energetic most of the time? Can you breathe easily when walking up a staircase of 20 steps? Do you feel physically comfortable wearing skinny jeans or body-hugging dresses? Physically comfortable means you can move freely in your body-hugging clothes without worrying about ripping materials apart in public.

Weight is an important indicator of our overall health condition. When you go to get an annual physical exam, the first number the medical staff measures is your weight. Another way to look at it is our overall health depends on how we manage our weight.

Key barriers to achieving our desired weight, health condition, and fitness goals include our physiology, mental health, nutrition, exercise, environmental factors, etc. Let's examine the key barriers that are common to all.

What Women Over 40 Need to Know - Physiology

Even if we keep the exact same lifestyles as we had in our 20s and 30s, women tend to gain weight after turning 40 and even more after turning 50, near menopause.

In layman's terms, as we get older, our body composition changes. As we age, our metabolism slows down, we lose muscle mass, and we experience hormonal changes, which all contribute to weight gain. Weight gain in turn causes breathing problems, heart and blood vessel disease, type 2 diabetes, which negatively affect the quality of our lives.

Even for naturally thin women, after they turn 40, they notice their belly fat starts showing more, and their waistlines increase each year. Again, the increase in our belly fat has much to do with our physiological changes after turning 40. As we age, our estrogen level drops, and estrogen seems to have an effect on where fat accumulates. Having a large amount of belly fat raises the risk of high blood pressure, heart disease, diabetes, certain cancers, stroke, fatty liver, etc.

Physiological changes lead to weight gain that leads to more health issues. More health issues can lead to reduced activity levels, which in turn can cause more weight gain. It becomes a negative feedback loop. You are one step closer to preventing or slowing down this negative feedback loop by being aware of our inevitable physiological changes.

What Women Over 40 Need to Know - Nutrition

According to a survey, the prevalence of diabetes and prediabetes among people aged 40–49 is 11.1% and 40.3%. The good news is prediabetes can be reversed through proper nutrition and weight management, such as reducing the intake of refined carbs (e.g., white rice, white bread, white pasta, etc.), added sugars (e.g., sugary beverages, cookies, cakes, candy, etc.), saturated and trans fats (e.g., butter, sausages, bacon, cheese, etc.).

Now, you probably think life would be so dull if I could not enjoy delicious food. Do not worry. This section is about increasing your awareness of the health impact of foods and drinks that taste good but lack the right kind of nutrition your body needs. We are living in the instant gratification era. Foods that tend to give us instant gratification, which we are so used to expecting, may also increase the risk of heart disease, prediabetes, type 2 diabetes, etc.

According to the World Bank data, in 2020, the average life expectancy of women in the United States is 77.28 years old. Is it better to let instant gratification permanently sabotage our health for the next 20 - 40 years, or do we exercise moderation to live a quality life over the next 20- 40 years? Most logical people would choose the latter.

Later in the book, I will share nutrition hacks that allow you to enjoy tasty foods while helping you lose weight.

What Women Over 40 Need to Know - Exercise

There are a lot of myths about exercising and staying active. Celebrity culture is so dominant in our society. We often see super-toned celebrities show clips of their hard-core exercise routines (e.g., intense cardio, pilates, weight lifting, etc.) on Instagram or talk about their dedication to fitness in interviews. Inevitably, most people think losing or managing weight requires a ton of exercise or long hours in the gym.

We are not celebrities. Most of us don't or shouldn't have to rely heavily on our physical appearance to make a living. Most American women over 40, working or stay-at-home moms, do not have the time or energy to spend more than 40 minutes in the gym daily. If we include the time it takes to drive, change clothes, and shower, total gym time can easily add up to 1 hour to 1.5 hours each day.

So, does that mean we can never be as lean as gym rats? Absolutely not. You will soon learn easy hacks to get you leaner and feel stronger without spending much time in the gym. I will put in layman's terms to explain why exercising more can have a diminishing return and why it might not be efficient to spend more time in the gym.

It is commonly known that weight loss is a result of creating a calorie deficit, meaning the number of calories you burn exceeds the number of calories you put in your body. The traditional belief is that exercise can help burn more calories and create a calorie deficit.

Many studies have shown that more exercise does not always burn more calories. Exercising more or longer does not proportionally result in weight loss and could even result in injuries. Since I promised in the introduction that I would not bore you with big scientific analyses, I will put this in layman's terms. The first 200 calories we burn through exercise matter the most, which can be achieved on a StairMaster in 10-15 minutes, depending on your setting. After that, calorie-burning might start to plateau. That is why there is no reason to become a gym rat.

In some cases, more exercise can cause people to eat more. As a matter of fact, I have a friend who was taking diet pills and swimming 1 hour each day. She found herself craving more food after each swimming session. The amount of exercise she was getting was counterproductive to her taking diet pills. She hardly lost any weight and started experiencing the side effects of her diet pills.

Exercise in moderation is great for our health and can certainly help manage or lose weight. Exercise is only a small portion of staying active. This book will discuss hacks to help you easily stay active and burn more calories outside the gym.

What Women Over 40 Need to Know - Mental Health

Maintaining mental health is critical to proper weight management. Mental health refers to our emotional, psychological and social well-being. Mental health is a broad category and takes commitment to condition our mental health. Why do we need to be more aware of our mental health? Mental health can impact our judgment, beliefs, and confidence needed to achieve goals in life. Mental health determines how we handle stress. And stress directly causes excessive belly fat and weight gain.

Women over 40 naturally have more responsibilities at home, work, or both until kids are gone or we retire. Naturally, we face more stressful circumstances when juggling family, relationships, work life, social pressure, etc.

Since I promised not to give big scientific analyses, I will summarize them in layman's terms. Stress triggers the body's cortisol, which is our body's main stress-fighting hormone. It works with certain parts of the brain to control our mood, motivation, fear, etc. Cortisol also helps control blood sugar levels, regulate metabolism, manage how the body uses nutrients, etc. When there is a high level of cortisol caused by stress, cortisol can throw other systems in our body out of balance.

It is common that we tend to eat excessively or grab those guilty pleasures the most when we feel stressed. That is the result of cortisol doing its work to fight stress. When under stress, we can feel instant gratification through increased cortisol and uncontrollable eating. We also end up increasing belly fat and gaining weight.

Just like physical health, mental health takes time and conscious efforts to achieve. I mention mental health here so you are aware of the direct relationship between stress management and weight management.

Although this book is not focused on mental health, it is so important to start developing a mental game, your belief system, as a critical part of your weight loss and weight management journey. The next chapter gives you simple hacks to help you strengthen your mental game.

Chapter 2: Your Belief System - Mental Hacks

One-Minute Daily Manifestation Exercises

First, you must believe you can achieve your weight loss and overall fitness goals. It is natural to feel unmotivated and even demoralized when fad diets, exercise, and diet pills do not give you the lasting results that you desire. After reading the previous chapter, you understand some key barriers to achieving your desired weight. And it is never late to learn new hacks.

Many people, even for those who seem to be very religious or spiritual, have a hard time believing in miracles until they see miracles happen in front of their eyes. Therefore, let's first work on your mental game - your belief system.

How often have you heard people say, "If I make X amount of money, I will buy a house." "If I achieve this career goal, I will get married and settle down." "If I meet the right person, I will have a committed relationship." "If I make and save enough, I will start traveling more." When people make these so-called goals or resolutions, they use conditional statements and describe their results in the future tense because deep down, they do not really believe these future goals can happen without meeting self-imposed conditions, meaning if I do X, then I will get Y. These self-imposed conditions are limiting beliefs that come from a place of lack. So, what ends up happening is that many people keep chasing their dreams for most of their lives. Some never achieve their goals.

This might not be intuitively obvious to you, especially if you have been taught that we must work hard in order to achieve x, y, and z in life. Having a good work ethic is necessary and respectable. But it makes a world of difference in the speed at which we achieve our goals, if we first develop a deep belief system before making plans and taking actions.

I do not intend to use this succinct book to teach the Law of Attraction details here. I will summarize for you why we need to practice the Law of Attraction daily. The Law of Attraction, in the simplest term, is what we think is what we attract. This means we must first believe that the outcome of our desire is already achieved so we can attract the desired outcome. Having a deep belief system attracts helpful forces and favorable circumstances beyond your imagination but can help you achieve goals much quicker. Having a deep belief system can help you work smarter, stay open minded, and take advantage of available resources.

Now, let's put the Law of Attraction in the context of manifesting your weight loss & fitness goals. Believe you have achieved your weight loss goals before you physically achieve them. To develop a belief system, you want to be realistically aggressive in stating your intention or desire. For example, you would love to lose 20 lbs next week, but we all know that is extremely unlikely. So, that does not help you develop your belief system. On the other hand, you can state your intention as following affirmations:

- I am losing weight and getting fit now.
- I am so happy that I am losing 20 lbs.
- I am so happy that I am wearing my skinny jeans again.

Note all these affirmation statements are written in the present tense, which shows a deep conviction that your desired outcome is happening now. There is no conditional statement in any of these. This is how you start building a deep belief system in yourself. You can compare your feelings by reading out loud these 2 sets of statements and see which ones make you feel more empowered.

1a. I am so happy that I am 20 lbs lighter. Or 1b. I will be so happy if I am 20 lbs lighter.

2a. I am 10 lbs lighter & feeling great! Or 2b. If I lose 10 lbs, then I will feel great.

It should be pretty obvious that 1a and 2a lift your spirit, make you smile, and boost your confidence because you are losing weight and feeling lighter now, not in the future. Let's translate what you just learned into actionable steps.

Step 1. State your intention - Write down your affirmation (one sentence) in a journal every day using the sample affirmations above or your own version. You want to write the one-sentence affirmation in your journal 1-3 times. This should only take 30 seconds to complete. If you really can't finish writing one sentence 3 times in 30 seconds, you can type the statement on your computer or your phone instead.

Step 2. Claim your results - Stand in front of your bathroom or bedroom mirror, look into the mirror, and state the same affirmation out loud 3 times every day. This should only take 15 seconds to complete.

Hack #1: Write down your affirmation in a journal and state your affirmation out loud in front of a mirror 3 times EVERYDAY for 28 consecutive days.

Why do I recommend doing these 2 steps for 28 consecutive days? For most people, after doing a new thing for 28 days straight, this new routine becomes a habitual routine. You will soon see positive changes to your belief system and confidence level while achieving your weight loss and fitness goals.

Showing gratitude is another important component of manifesting your desired outcome. Instead of waiting to see results and then giving thanks in the future, you want to express gratitude now. You want to express gratitude daily as if you have already achieved the results.

Step 3. Express gratitude mentally or verbally 3 times every day, feel grateful, and get excited about achieving your goals while expressing gratitude. This should take no more than 15 seconds to complete.

You want to do this during your morning affirmation / journaling routine. You can express gratitude again throughout the day or before you go to bed. Again, make sure you express gratitude in the present tense. Below are some examples of expressing your gratitude:

- I am so grateful for effortlessly losing weight.
- I am so grateful for feeling lighter and thinner now.
- I am so thankful for my new healthy lifestyle.

These are just examples you can use immediately or as inspirations to create your own version. When you express gratitude, try to feel excited about receiving the desired outcome. When you add positive emotions to your gratitude statement, you reinforce your belief system even more.

Hack #2: Repeat your gratitude statement mentally or verbally 3 times EVERYDAY for 28 consecutive days; feel grateful and excited while expressing gratitude.

You might ask how can I feel excited when I have not seen much change in my weight yet. Again, Hack #2 is about strengthening your inner game and helping you develop your belief system, so you can achieve your goals and achieve them sooner. You have nothing to lose by thinking positively and believing in yourself. However, if you keep dwelling on the negative aspects of your life, you will end up attracting negative circumstances, according to the Law of Attraction.

Manifesting Accountability Tracking

Hack #1 and #2 include 3 simple steps that only take ONE MINUTE for you to do every day. You must do all three steps for at least 28 consecutive days until they become your daily ritual.

Below are sample tracking charts to help you take accountability during the first 28 days. No matter how busy or how scattered you are, do Hack #1 and #2 the first thing after you wake up, so you will not forget. And these 3 steps will help you feel confident and empowered all day long.

It is okay if you forget to write down or verbalize you affirmation once or twice the first week. But make sure you do ALL 3 steps daily during the following 3 weeks. It takes only one minute to complete the mental exercises. There is no excuse for not doing them.

1 Minute Daily Manifestation - Day 1 - Day 7	Mon	Tue	Wed	Thu	Fri	Sat	Sun
Step 1). Did you write down your weightloss affirmation statement? - 30 seconds	Y	Y	N	Y	Y	Y	Y
Step 2). Did you look into the mirror and state the same weight loss affirmation you wrote out loud 3 times? - 15 seconds	Y	Y	Y	Y	N	Y	Y
Step 3). Did you say your gratitude statement mentally or verbally while feeling grateful and excited 3 times? - 15 seconds	Y	Y	Y	Y	Y	Y	Y

1 Minute Daily Manifestation - Day 8 - Day 14	Mon	Tue	Wed	Thu	Fri	Sat	Sun
Step 1). Did you write down your weightloss affirmation statement? - 30 seconds	Y	Y	Y	Y	Y	Y	Y
Step 2). Did you look into the mirror and state the same weight loss affirmation you wrote out loud 3 times? - 15 seconds	Y	Y	Y	Y	Y	Y	Y
Step 3). Did you say your gratitude statement mentally or verbally while feeling grateful and excited 3 times? - 15 seconds	Y	Y	Y	Y	Y	Y	Y

1 Minute Daily Manifestation - Day 15 - Day 21	Mon	Tue	Wed	Thu	Fri	Sat	Sun
Step 1). Did you write down your weightloss affirmation statement? - 30 seconds	Y	Y	Y	Y	Y	Y	Y
Step 2). Did you look into the mirror and state the same weight loss affirmation you wrote out loud 3 times? - 15 seconds	Y	Y	Y	Y	Y	Y	Y
Step 3). Did you say your gratitude statement mentally or verbally while feeling grateful and excited 3 times? - 15 seconds	Y	Y	Y	Y	Y	Y	Y

1 Minute Daily Manifestation - Day 22 - Day 28	Mon	Tue	Wed	Thu	Fri	Sat	Sun
Step 1). Did you write down your weightloss affirmation statement? - 30 seconds	Y	Y	Y	Y	Y	Y	Y
Step 2). Did you look into the mirror and state the same weight loss affirmation you wrote out loud 3 times? - 15 seconds	Y	Y	Y	Y	Y	Y	Y
Step 3). Did you say your gratitude statement mentally or verbally while feeling grateful and excited 3 times? - 15 seconds	Y	Y	Y	Y	Y	Y	Y

You can use a printed calendar or a magnet calendar that you can stick on your fridge to track your 1-minute daily manifestation exercises over the next 4 weeks. You want to put the calendar for tracking in a very visible place, such that it is impossible for you not to see it every day. You will feel great each time you write a check mark or a Y for yes.

Manifesting Results by Taking Inspired Actions

As you strengthen your inner game and develop your belief system for losing X lbs and achieving your overall fitness goals (e.g., lower BMI or blood pressure to the healthy range, etc.), you have to take inspired actions such as applying the hacks that you will learn in the following sections of the book to manifest results. Manifesting is not about meditating or daydreaming for hours without taking any action in the physical world.

How can you tell the difference between actions vs. inspired actions? When actions do not inspire you, you will feel some resistance, and you do not get excited about them. For example, accepting a lower-paying job to pay bills is a common action many people take and feel disappointed, because this action comes from a place of fear and lack. On the contrary, politely suggesting a reasonably higher pay rate backed by compelling reasons to the hiring manager is an inspired action, which comes from a place of belief, strength and abundance.

Inspired actions tend to give you hope or excitement, and they are not difficult for you to take. When you feel inspired, you won't even see these actions as hard work. New ideas, hints, and recommendations do not just coincidentally pop up. Remember, your new belief system helps you attract solutions to you. When the solutions are presented to you, you need to take inspired actions now.

Hack #3: Do not procrastinate. Take inspired actions by applying hacks listed in the following sections, starting TODAY.

The sooner you take inspired actions, the sooner you achieve your goals. Although it only takes 1 minute every day to complete these mental hacks, this chapter likely takes more mental processing than the rest of the book for some readers because it involves reprogramming their thought processes. Developing a deep belief system might be challenging for some people, especially if they have been exposed to limiting beliefs for too long (e.g., our body starts going downhill after age 40, anti-aging must cost a lot of money, etc.). Getting mentally conditioned at the beginning of each day is critical if you want to achieve results in a shorter amount of time.

Chapter 3: Simple Nutrition Hacks - Morning

You are reading this book because you intend to lose weight. So, let's not beat around the bush. Let's get your weight number daily before drinking and eating anything. This might sound dreadful. We cannot make progress if we hold onto fear.

Treat weight measurement as a simple tracking routine to help you stay focused and stay on track. When you see your weight start going down even by half a pound, you will love doing weight measurements every day.

The reason we want to measure before taking any food or water is because you actually weigh the least in the morning, especially after you did number 1 and number 2 in the bathroom. Our weight can increase by 2-3 lbs as we eat 3 meals and snacks and drink 8 glasses of water. We want to make sure the measurement is roughly taken around the same time each day. For women who are still menstruating, do not panic if you see weight gain (as much as 3 lbs) due to water retention. After your period is over, your weight will come down.

Weighing yourself before your day starts serves as a gentle reminder to apply the hacks you learned in this book every day. Please do not get frustrated or give up, if you do not see your weight come down every week. Even if your weight does not change immediately, you are still on the path to becoming a healthier version of yourself. Also, do not get cocky if you see your weight drop 2-3 lbs in 24 hours, and stop applying the hacks for a few days. It might take some people as quickly as 24 - 48 hours to drop 3 lbs because the hacks discussed in this book help them lose water weight or move wastes out of the body quicker. But you still have to keep creating a calorie deficit daily to lose fat, especially the stubborn belly fat, and keep weight off.

Hack #4: Weigh yourself <u>every</u> morning before drinking and eating.

Starving oneself is not the way to lose weight and can often cause people to overeat later. We need to use healthy and sustainable methods to create a calorie deficit to lose fat. As mentioned in the previous section, exercise can only help you burn so many calories per day. How many calories we consume can directly impact how quickly we can create a calorie deficit.

Why do we often consume more calories than the body really needs? It could be caused by stress, low blood sugar levels, lack of quality nutrients, or confusing hunger with something else, such as dehydration. Because some of the symptoms of dehydration can resemble symptoms of hunger (e.g., fatigue, lightheadedness), let's make sure your body does not confuse thirst and hunger, which can cause you to overeat.

When you first wake up, after you weigh yourself, you need to drink water first, preferably warm water, not cold water, not coffee or juice. Drinking warm water can kick-start your metabolism. Keeping yourself hydrated can help prevent your brain from confusing dehydration with hunger; therefore, you will be less tempted to grab high-calorie foods such as donuts or bagels in front of you at home or at work.

Vinegar has many health benefits, including supporting weight loss. Taking vinegar directly is torture, but you can take apple cider vinegar capsules instead. That way you cannot taste anything sour. Apple cider vinegar contains acetic acid, which is known to reduce the absorption of carbohydrates, causes the body to burn more fat and helps provide a feeling of fullness.

You can easily find apple cider vinegar capsules on Amazon. Make sure you read the reviews and try to purchase the brands with plenty of reviews with an average of 4.3-star rating and above.

Hack #5a: Take apple cider vinegar capsules (quantity should be based on directions printed by the brand) with a glass of warm water <u>daily</u> after you weigh yourself before eating anything.

There are scientific studies on the benefits of drinking lemon water in the morning, such as boosting your energy & alertness, getting more bowel movements, etc. If you like to drink acidic water, you can drink fresh lemon water as an alternative.

You can simply hand-squeeze half of a lemon into a glass of warm water. Depending on where you live, the cost of a bottle of apple cider vinegar capsules that typically lasts 30 days might be similar to the cost of buying fresh lemons.

Hack #5b: Alternatively, drink a glass of warm, fresh lemon water <u>daily</u>, after you weigh yourself before eating anything.

Please do not buy lemon juice in cartons, then pour it into a glass of warm water. Lemon juice or lemonade sold in stores contains added sugar. The warm water mentioned in Hack #5a and #5b should have zero added sugar. Make sure you apply either hack #5a (preferred) or #5b each morning if you really like lemon to help you stay hydrated, feel fuller, and boost your energy.

For those of you who must have coffee in the morning to get your day going, let's make sure you still get the caffeine you crave but with less calorie intake. If you take coffee black, you don't need to tweak anything. But if you drink coffee with cream and sugar or you are a latte drinker, you need to replace cream/milk & sugar with low-calorie plant- based milk. For example, unsweetened almond milk contains plant-based protein, calcium, vitamin D, and zinc with zero added sugar. Milk, on the other hand, easily contains 12 grams of sugar per cup regardless of fat %.

Hack #6: Replace cream/milk & sugar in your coffee with low-calorie plant-based milk to get a great flavor while reducing calorie intake.

There are quite a few types of plant-based milk. I mentioned almond milk here because you can easily get unsweetened almond milk from grocery stores, and most coffee shops these days have almond milk. Almond milk has a more neutral flavor, and it is less sweet than coconut milk and oat milk.

Next, we need to feed the body with high-quality energy foods. The human body needs essential dietary fats to support cell function, protect our organs, give us energy, and keep us warm. We do not want to consume too much fat, which leads to weight gain and health issues. On a typical food label, you can see Total Fat,

Saturated Fat and Trans Fat on the top. The reason labels are required to explicitly show the amount of saturated fat and transfat per serving is because consuming too much of these two types dietary fats can cause health issues (e.g., heart disease, stroke).

Since this book is about making healthy tweaks, I will not list all the scientific discoveries about each type of fat here. Let's focus on the key concept you need to grasp and actionable steps you can easily take now.

Among all the dietary fat types, we want to increase unsaturated fats intake, still in moderation, and try to lower saturated and trans fats intake.

Foods that contain high **saturated** fats include dairy products (e.g., butter, cheese, milk, ice cream), fatty cuts of meat, sausages, cured meats, cream, coconut milk, coconut oil, palm oil, etc.

Foods that contain high **unsaturated** fats include nuts, seeds, nut butter, avocado, fish, olive, etc. For most people, there is no time to cook fish in the morning, but once in a while, you can get smoked salmon from wholesale stores (e.g., Costco) that is ready to eat and more affordable if you are not allergic to fish.

Hack #7: Consume 1 serving of foods high in unsaturated fats and low in carbs in the morning <u>daily</u>.

Next, let's talk about the types of carbs you can consume in the morning. We want to reduce the intake of refined carbs and added sugar, such as white bread, bagels, donuts, pancakes & waffles made with white flour, cereal, pre-packaged breakfast bars, etc. Don't worry; you will not starve by reducing your intake of refined carbs and added sugar, especially if you have already completed the hacks mentioned above.

If you have to have a slice of bread in the morning, then make an avocado toast or nut butter toast using one slice of whole-grain bread. On the nutrition label, whole wheat bread might show a similar or slightly lower amount of carbs and calories as white bread, but you get a lot more fiber from whole-grain bread. Fiber can boost metabolism, increase bowel movements, help control blood sugar levels and make us feel fuller.

Another comfort food many Americans grow up eating is cereal with milk. While cereals contain a good amount of vitamins and minerals, they are also high in carbs (including added sugar) and relatively low in protein and unsaturated fat. That is why people often feel hungry mid-morning after eating cereal. Try to eat whole-grain cereals with more fiber instead.

Also, when eating cereals, you can replace cow milk that is high in added sugar (carbs) with unsweetened almond milk to reduce overall calorie consumption as mentioned in Hack #6.

You still can have some form of instant gratification by having fresh fruits in the morning to get vitamins and minerals and give you a sugar boost without consuming added sugar. Fruit juices that come in cartons and bottles sold in stores usually contain added sugar.

Hack #8: Reduce or avoid refined carbs and fruit juices that contain added sugar. Eat whole grains and/or fresh fruits instead for more quality nutrients.

Morning Routine and Strategy Summary:

Let's put what you learned from the last chapter (mental hacks) and this chapter (morning hacks) together; our daily morning routine with strategic hacks includes:

- Get mentally conditioned (1 minute manifestation exercises)
- Check weight
- Get hydrated and curb appetite (warm water with apple cider vinegar capsules or fresh lemon)
- Energize the body with quality nutrients (high in unsaturated fats, fiber, vitamins, minerals and low in carbs) and keep the body feel full

Chapter 4: Simple Nutrition Hacks - Mid-Day

This chapter shows how you can have a healthy and delicious meal without feeling hungry. If you can work from home, pack your lunch, or make your own salad at work, you can use the hacks below to easily make a lunch salad to let your body get plenty of nutrients and feel full without consuming a lot of calories.

To make a nutrient-rich, tasty, and low-calorie lunch salad, you need these 3 essential categories: leafy greens, lean protein(s), and low-calorie salad dressing.

First, we need leafy greens (e.g., arugula, mixed greens) that are rich in nutrients, low in calories, and can help us feel full. Leafy green vegetables, such as arugula, contain a good amount of dietary fiber, vitamins, and minerals the body needs. Consuming dietary fiber is essential to managing weight, lowering bad cholesterol to reduce heart disease risks, slowing down the absorption of sugar to reduce diabetes risks, and keeping the gut healthy by helping wastes move smoothly through the body. According to some studies, most Americans do not consume adequate amounts of dietary fiber the body needs. Nowadays, you can buy one lb of prewashed, organic baby arugula or mixed greens for $7 or less from big chain grocery stores. One lb of such greens can easily last 6 meals, so getting this type of leafy greens ready to eat is very economical and time-efficient.

Then, we add lean proteins, such as boiled eggs, grilled chicken, salmon, etc., that contain plenty of nutrients the body needs and can give us energy and help us feel full. If you are on a budget or do not like to cook, boil 8-10 eggs on Sunday, put them in the fridge, and on each consecutive day, slice 2 boiled eggs and put them in the salad. That is the quickest and perhaps the most economical way to make a nutritious lunch salad.

To make your salad enjoyable, your salad dressing plays a big part in the flavor. Then, you will want to use your favorite vinaigrette dressing. The common theme with morning Hack #5a and #5b is consuming a small amount of acid, which helps regulate our blood sugar and helps us feel fuller.

To add more texture and nutrients to your salad, you can add high-protein nuts or seeds, such as walnuts, almonds, sunflower seeds, and flax seeds, if you are not allergic to them. If you have more time, you are welcome to add low-sugar fruits such as cherry tomatoes, berries, and avocados. As you may know, avocados are high in unsaturated fats, which can give us energy and help us feel full.

If you are a vegetarian, use your favorite plant-based proteins with your leafy salads.

Hack #9: Eat a leafy green salad with lean proteins and use a vinaigrette dressing 5 days each week.

Some of you might think I can not enjoy my salad without cheese. Yes, you can! Your body does not naturally crave cheese. If you follow the simple recipe listed in this chapter, the salad gives your body more nutrients than cheese; it tastes delicious, energizes you, and makes you feel full, and you do not need additional dairy ingredients such as cheese. Just try Hack #9 for a few days, and you will realize your body is satisfied with the leafy green salad without cheese.

If you do not get to eat lunch at home or you cannot make your salad at work, then try to eat leafy green salads with lean proteins as often as possible when eating out. And you can tell restaurant servers what ingredients to leave out (e.g., cheese, bacon, etc.). I have done that every single time, and not once any server rolled their eyes at me. But if the type of restaurants you frequent do not serve salads at all, then you can simply make and eat your leafy green salad for dinner. The bottom line is that when you eat a leafy green salad, according to Hack #9, either for lunch or dinner for at least 5 days each week, you will feel leaner and more energetic as soon as the 1st week. You can have one or two cheat days for those of you who were never into salads.

Hack #10: If you are a sandwich person, try peeling half of the sandwich bread off to reduce your carbs intake during lunch.

You will actually feel more energetic and more alert with less carbs intake.

If you really still feel hungry after a big bowl of leafy greens mixed with lean proteins, you can drink low-calorie soups during lunch, especially when you have more time to prepare your lunch on weekends.

Soup in this context can be lightly flavored liquids, such as miso soup, chicken broth (reduced sodium), beef stew, fish soup, etc. Why does the soup have to be low in sodium? Our body tends to retain more water if we eat salty foods.

Hack #11: Drink low-sodium and low-calorie soups, in addition to eating the leafy green salad with lean proteins if you have more time or do not feel full.

Below are examples of what your nutritious and tasty lunch could look like by applying these hacks, from the most basic combination to the more flavorful versions. You are welcome to add other ingredients that have quality nutrients (e.g., avocado, mushroom, peppers, etc.). For vegetarians, as mentioned above, you simply replace lean meat proteins with your favorite plant-based proteins.

Lunch salad examples:

- Leafy greens + lean proteins + vinaigrette dressing
- Leafy greens + lean proteins + nuts / seeds + vinaigrette dressing
- Leafy greens + lean proteins + nuts / seeds + low sugar fruits + vinaigrette dressing

Optional: Add a low-sodium & low-calorie soup (clear broth preferred), if you do not feel full after eating a salad.

The lunch hacks mentioned here are simple, budget-friendly, and sustainable hacks that you can apply immediately or use them as sources of inspiration. You can create your own combination of leafy greens, proteins, fruits, and flavors. The bottom line is that we want to consume high-quality nutrients, lower overall calorie intake, feel full and energized at the same time.

Chapter 5: Simple Nutrition Hacks - Afternoon

Many of us need to snack on some things in the afternoon due to work stress, boredom, old habits, or an actual calorie deficit. You can enjoy a healthy and delicious snack without consuming too many calories.

Chapter 4 (morning hacks) mentioned our body might confuse dehydration and hunger. By the time we feel thirsty, we are already dehydrated. Drinking water before snacking can help us stay hydrated and suppress appetite.

Hack #12: Drink water before snacking in the afternoon to stay hydrated and curb your appetite.

This is the only time of the entire day I recommend you count calories because 1). It is very easy to count the calories of a snack; 2). Make sure you get an energy boost without consuming excessive calories, so you will have the energy to stay physically active after work and before dinner; 3). Prevent you from binge eating at dinner time. Let's make wise choices and keep the total calorie consumption of the afternoon snack under 300 calories.

Hack #13: Eat fruits and/or nuts to get more nutrients and feel full. Try to keep the total calorie intake under 300 calories.

You can eat fruits like oranges, apples, pears, berries, and watermelon to get vitamins and minerals and help you stay hydrated. You do not want to overeat fruits, either. They taste good because they all contain some sugar, just not artificially added sugar. According to USDA, on average, 1 small orange has ~45 calories, 9 grams of sugar, and 1 medium-sized apple has ~95 calories, 19 grams of sugar. Eating 1 whole apple is totally fine, just don't try to inhale 3 apples.

One serving of honey-roasted peanuts has ~150 calories. If you eat nuts, try to eat nuts by themselves, not trail mix with added sugar from the vending machine. Granola bars do not make the cut here. They are highly processed with added sugar.

Since your afternoon snack time is likely just 2-3 hours after your lunch, you should feel full and energized if you consume 1 medium-sized apple + 1 serving of roasted peanuts = 245 calories or 2 small oranges + 1 serving of roasted peanuts = 240 calories.

If you cannot cut out your sugary candy, then eat a piece of dark chocolate. Dark chocolate is rich in nutrients, which can also help curb hunger.

Hack #14: If you have to have candy, eat a piece of dark chocolate instead. Try to keep the total calorie intake under 300 calories.

If you are not particularly fond of fruits or plain nuts, you can consume some nut butter or cream cheese to consume fats in moderation and curb hunger.

Hack #15: Eat 1 or 2 spoons of peanut butter, almond butter, or cream cheese to boost energy and curb hunger. Try to keep the total calorie intake under 300 calories.

Remember, we want to be strategic about consuming foods that give us energy and nutrients and make us feel full while reducing our overall calorie consumption.

And if you also drink coffee in the afternoon, remember to apply Hack #6: try to use low- sugar plant-based milk (e.g., unsweetened almond milk) to replace cream, sugar, and milk.

Chapter 6: Simple Nutrition Hacks - Evening

Most people who work or take care of the household during the day are less physically active after dinner. So, it is important that you stop eating after 7pm or 8pm at the latest, whether you go to bed at 9pm, 10pm, or midnight.

Some might wonder, what if I exercise at night to burn off what I eat after 8pm? Yes, you can, but it is not practical or sustainable for most people to do intense exercises after a busy day and after dinner. I will talk about doing some mild movements in the evening to help your body burn more calories later in this book, but by no means, any of those hacks is physically intensive. Plus, you want to take it easy in the evening and avoid getting your body all worked up such that you cannot easily fall asleep at night. Chapter 12 talks about getting a good night's sleep, which can also help you lose weight and keep weight off.

Hack #16: Stop eating after 8pm at least 5 days every week.

Some of you might ask, what if I have to attend social gatherings that tend to serve dinner late? Well, Hack #16 gives you some wiggle room. I am happy for you if you have a very active social life. You can have a couple of cheat days, or you can eat dinner at home before you go out. At social gatherings, you can nibble on some low-calorie foods to blend in without eating a full meal later than 8pm. Remember, this book is intended to help you make strategic and incremental adjustments to your lifestyle to lose weight and keep weight off.

Next, let's talk about how to reduce weight gain due to water retention, although it is temporary for people who do not have underlying healthy issues. The human body is made up of over 70% water. Drinking enough water is essential to our health. However, excessive water retention makes us feel bloated and look swollen. Persistent water retention can be a sign of underlying health issues. You should consult your doctor if you consistently experience water retention. But if you are generally healthy and you suddenly see 3-10 lbs of weight gain in a short amount of time, it could be caused by water retention. You can reduce or prevent water retention by eating low-sodium and low-carb foods for dinner.

If you eat salty foods all the time, your taste buds become so desensitized that you do not even realize how salty is salty and how much excess sodium you consume that causes water retention. Your food will not taste bland when you reduce the amount of salt in your food by 25% or replace regular soy sauce with low-sodium soy sauce for a stir-fry dish. You can reprogram your taste buds to get used to low-sodium foods if you consistently reduce your salt intake by 25% for several weeks. Low-sodium foods will start to taste more flavorful to you over time.

On most days each week, you also want to consume less starchy foods (e.g., potatoes, bread, rice, pasta, etc.) for dinner. Starchy foods cause the body to retain water as well.

Hack #17: Eat low-sodium and less starchy foods for dinner to avoid water retention at least 5 days every week.

Let's incrementally reduce or replace less healthy ingredients, such as refined carbs, to make this weight loss journey enjoyable and sustainable. Refined carbs are lower in nutrients and can cause spikes in blood sugar levels, leading to overeating. Refined carbs refer to white rice, white bread, white pasta, pastries made with white flour, sugars, and sweetened beverages. Many studies have shown that the consumption of refined carbohydrates can result in obesity and type 2 diabetes.

If you frequently eat rice in the evening, I am not suggesting you completely stop eating rice. There is an alternative to white rice. You might be pleasantly surprised that brown rice has a more interesting texture and flavor than white rice. Brown rice is minimally processed, and it has more fiber and fewer calories than white rice.

If you frequently eat pasta in the evening, I am not suggesting you completely stop eating pasta either. You can eat pasta made with whole grains instead. When you put sauce on your pasta, are you really going to tell the big flavor difference between white pasta vs. whole wheat pasta?!

Even after you replace refined carbs with minimally processed carbs, let's try to cut your total carbs intake by 50% and increase your intake of lean proteins and vegetables during dinner.

Hack #18: Reduce or minimize refined carbs for dinner to avoid spikes in blood sugar levels that cause overeating; cut total carbs intake by 50%; increase proportions of lean proteins and vegetables.

The strategy here is to make tweaks to what you eat during dinner so you can gradually and willingly reduce or avoid high-calorie foods that are relatively lower in nutrients. You can have carbs for dinner, but you can replace refined carbs with better carbs and reduce your total consumption of carbs without feeling hungry.

Let's talk about the essential nutrients you can consume for dinner while making good choices. Below are different combination examples:

Proteins + Vegetables

- Lean proteins - chicken, lean beef or pork cuts, seafood, tofu, eggs, etc.
- Vegetables - at least one green vegetable that contains a good amount of fiber, vitamins, and minerals (e.g., green bean, spinach, bok choy, celery, etc.)

Proteins + Vegetables + Fruits (as dessert)

Lean proteins - chicken, lean beef or pork, seafood, tofu, eggs, etc.
- Vegetables - at least one green vegetable that contains a good amount of fiber, vitamins, and minerals
- Optional - eat fruit as dessert; recommend oranges or berries with less sugar.

Proteins + Vegetables + Carbs (reduce your normal portion by 50%)

- Lean proteins - chicken, lean beef or pork, seafood, tofu, eggs, etc.
- Vegetables - at least one green vegetable that contains a good amount of fiber, vitamins, and minerals
- Carbs (cut your normal dinner serving size by 50%) - potatoes, sweet potatoes, brown rice, whole wheat pasta, etc.

For flavors, be sure to use condiments that are low in sodium (e.g., less salt, low-sodium soy sauce), non-dairy (e.g., use safflower and olive oil instead of butter), less sugary, and less spicy.

Again, the approach is not about making your dinner tasteless; it is about eating everything in moderation by making incremental reductions.

If you have applied 70% of the hacks #1-#18, you will not feel hungry or attempt to overeat at night. If you ever feel tempted to chow down bread or eat ice cream after 8pm, then repeat the mental hacks - stand in front of a mirror and say your affirmation out loud 3 times - "I am happily losing weight now!" You can reprogram your brain to focus on happy results instead of hungry feelings.

Chapter 7: Easy Hacks to Burn More Calories - At Gym

How to Work Out in the Gym Less and Achieve Greater Results

For those of you who do not like to go to the gym, you will be happy to know that you do not have to become a gym rat to lose weight. For those of you who like to work out in the gym and do not have more time to spend at the gym, the good news is that you can lose weight with less time spent in the gym.

You can squeeze in a quality cardio workout in the gym in 30 min. Burning the first 200 calories is critical, which does not take too much time to achieve this. This can be accomplished on a treadmill under 30 minutes or on a StairMaster under 20 minutes if the settings are moderate or a bit intense. But if you have heart or joint issues, you should always consult a doctor first before doing any moderate to intense workout.

By the way, when I say 20~30 minutes, it means actual workout time (excluding break time). A quality 20~30-minute workout session can easily burn 150-200 calories.

Hack #19: Gym workout - less is more; do a short and quality workout session to burn 200+ calories, 3~5 times a week.

During each workout session, you will want to adjust the speed and intensity when you only use one machine or the same set of machines to trick your body. If you keep working on the same muscle group with the same intensity every day, your body will get used to it. You can manually adjust your favorite cardio machines or use pre-programmed settings such as climbing a hill, where there is a variation in speed and resistance level during your workout.

For those of you who do not like to work out, you can start by doing something mild on a treadmill, where you can adjust the speed and inclination angle. Then, you can switch to a StairMaster. Or you can alternate between the treadmill and

StairMaster in the same workout session.

An example of a 30-minute treadmill workout in week 1:

- First 5 minutes, set inclination angle = 5 and speed = 3.0
- Next 10 minutes, set inclination angle = 7 and speed = 3.2
- Next 10 minutes, option 1. set inclination angle = 8 and speed = 3.0 (if you want more resistance at a slower pace) or option 2. set inclination angle = 8 and speed = 3.3 (if you can handle more resistance and a faster pace)
- Last 5 minutes, set inclination angle = 3 and speed = 2.5 to cool down

A combo example during a 30-minute workout in week 2:

Spend 15 minutes on a treadmill

- First 5 minutes, set inclination angle = 6 and speed = 3.2
- Next 5 minutes, set inclination angle = 8 and speed = 3.4
- Last 5 minutes, set inclination angle = 5 and speed = 3.0

Spend 15 minutes on a StairMaster, select the climbing hill option

- First 5 minutes, set level = 6
- Next 5 minutes, set level = 8 to increase resistance
- Last 5 minutes, set level = 5 to cool down

Let's say that you are traveling or super busy in week 3 and you only have 20 minutes for a workout session.

An example of a 20-minute workout session:

Spend 15 minutes on a StairMaster, select the climbing hill option

- First 5 minutes, set level = 8
- Next 5 minutes, set level = 10 to increase resistance
- Last 5 minutes, set level = 6 to cool down

Spend next 5 minutes on a rowing machine to work on your upper body and core.

These are just examples for illustration purposes to show how you can vary resistance and speed to get the maximum results in a short amount of time by preventing your body from getting used to the exercise settings and preventing your metabolic rate from plateauing. You should adjust the settings that incrementally push your limit without causing discomfort or injuries. For those of you who have existing health conditions, please consult your doctor before doing any intense cardio exercise.

Hack #20: Gym workout - vary resistance and speed during each workout session.

If you need more motivation, you can join group classes. These classes are often 1 hour long. As Hack #19 mentioned, you do not need to stay there for the full hour unless you have the time and enjoy staying longer.

Hack #21: Gym workout - attend group classes to get motivated and keep workout time 30 minutes.

This book is about sharing simple and practical hacks that are easy and sustainable for you. There are many great machines in the gym that can work on different parts of your body. There are plenty of workout books that talk about lifting weights that can burn more calories. Well, they can also cause muscle injuries and need longer break time in between sets.

I will not go into gory details about every single machine in the gym that you should try. Hack #19 - #20 are the lowest-hanging fruits that you can pick, starting today. Everyone knows how to walk, and everyone knows how to climb stairs. We focus on walking and climbing more strategically to start melting fat off your body. Once you are more self-motivated to go to the gym, you can create all kinds of workout combinations that suit you.

After working out, some people feel full, while others might feel hungry pretty soon after. We do not want to experience hunger because that can lead to binge eating at the next meal. Make sure you drink at least 12-16 oz of water post-workout to replenish water and curb your appetite.

Hack #22: Drink plenty of water post-workout to curb hunger before the next meal.

Chapter 8: Easy Hacks to Burn More Calories - Outdoor

Burning calories is not limited by location and equipment. You can have fun while being outside. Whether it is playing tennis, pickleball, golf, softball, hiking, or swimming, as long as you keep your body moving, you are burning some calories. When you are having fun, you end up burning calories without even trying.

You do not need to keep score when playing sports to get all stressed out. Keeping your body moving and having fun at the same time is winning half of your weight loss battle. Having partners join you can motivate you to keep moving. Being active outside is good for the mind and body.

For busy moms, you might wonder how do I find time? Remember, your child learns from you. If you stay active and engage in a fun outdoor activity, your child will likely act the same. You want to stay active for you and your child. So, make time to play a sport or participate in an outdoor activity with your family and friends.

And when you go watch your children play sports, try to stand (without blocking other people's views) as much as possible and move your legs.

For single women, there are outdoor activity-related group meetups that can be fun for you to join if you cannot find any friends to play pickleball or tennis with you.

For those of you who have space for gardening, you can easily burn more calories through lifting, bending down, getting up, walking, digging, mowing, cutting, etc. Instead of admiring your neighbor's blooming roses, try to grow some flowers yourself while losing weight, even if you do not have a good track record of keeping plants alive. By the way, gardening can be quite therapeutic.

Hack #23: Engage in a fun outdoor activity that keeps you moving for at least 30 minutes twice a week.

Why do I recommend doing a fun outdoor activity at least twice a week? In case you do not feel like going to the gym 5 days a week, you can substitute outdoor activities for 1 or 2 gym workout sessions

Chapter 9: Easy Hacks to Burn More Calories - At Home

You Can Easily Burn More Calories at Home

As mentioned in Chapter 1, exercise only burns a relatively small amount of calories. You spend more time at home than at the gym, and you can keep burning calories at home.

If you do not have joint issues, standing is generally healthier than sitting. So, you want to increase the amount of time you stand on your feet while you are at home.

If you work from home or spend several hours a week on the computer in your home office, you can purchase an adjustable standing desk from Amazon for between $100 - $200. Standing while you are working has a lot of benefits, including burning more calories and reducing muscle/tendon stiffness.

As a matter of fact, if it is not physically uncomfortable for you to stand and eat at the same time, then you can stand while you eat! Studies have shown combining standing and eating can speed up digestion and your body's metabolism of food. When you help your children with homework, you can alternate standing and sitting.

Hack #24: Increase standing time at home daily.

For those of you who work in the service industry and already stand more than 5 hours at work each day, you just want to go home and sit down. There is a way to burn more calories while sitting. You can keep moving your legs, lift your heels up and drop them, and gently sway your legs from side to side. And you can tell others in the room that you do not have restless leg syndrome!

Hack #25: Move or fidget your legs while sitting as often as you can.

You can take a 15-20 min walk in a safe area after dinner at least 4 times each week. You can walk in circles in your living area or your own yard. You do not want to sit on the couch or lay down right after dinner, which can easily accumulate fat. You also do not want to do intense cardio after dinner. Taking a 20-min leisurely walk after dinner is beneficial to your health.

Hack #26: Take a 15-20 min walk after dinner as often as you can.

If you have stairs inside the home or a few steps out on the front porch, try to go up and down the steps for 5-10 minutes after dinner. Walking up and down stairs burns more calories than walking on a flat surface at a moderate pace. Walking up and down stairs can improve your cardio fitness and muscle strength.

Hack #27: Walk up and down stairs (if you have them at home) for 5-10 minutes after dinner as often as you can.

If you have joint pain or don't have stairs, then stick to Hack #26. **You will want to double the duration of doing Hack #26 or #27, if you did not exercise or engage in any outdoor activity at all during the day.**

When watching your favorite shows or listening to music or podcasts, you can do sit ups and push-ups at a slow pace. **You can do the lazy style sit-ups or the easy-style push-ups. The bottom line is keeping your body moving at a comfortable pace, while consuming media content.** You will not even feel that you are doing much work when you are mostly focused on media content consumption. Even if you take a 10 seconds break between sit-ups, you can easily complete 4 sit ups per minute and 50 sit-ups in less than 13 minutes.

Hack #28: Do sit-ups and push-ups while consuming media content (e.g., TV, music, podcast) at least 3 times each week.

Cleaning and tidying up your home can burn calories; whether you are vacuuming, mopping, or wiping, different parts of your body are moving. It is one stone shooting two birds - burning calories and keeping your place clean and organized.

Some urban households with financial means choose to use maid cleaning services. You can still use those services once a month for deep cleaning. Try to spend at least 30 minutes each week cleaning and/or organizing your home.

Hack #29: Clean and organize your home more often!

Chapter 10: Easy Hacks to Burn More Calories - At Work

You Can Easily Burn More Calories at Work

When we are awake, we often spend more time at work than elsewhere. For desk worker bees, there are a number of ways to burn more calories at work without using any equipment.

If you work inside a building, use the stairs in the building to burn calories. If your office happens to be on the first floor, you can still walk up and down the stairs for 5 minutes after lunch.

Hack #30: Skip the elevator and take the stairs.

Many workplaces, even public schools, provide employees with standing desks. Plus, many employers do reimburse ergonomic equipment purchases. If you can order an adjustable standing desk at work, definitely do so. If you don't have any physical discomfort while standing, try to stand for as long as possible while you are at work. It helps relieve muscle pain and burn more calories than sitting.

Hack #31: Stand for as long as possible while you are on your computer.

Any chance you can get to walk from your desk to a conference room or bathroom, try to speed walk. Speed walking can burn more calories, and it can have a secondary benefit to you. Your boss and colleagues might perceive you as someone who is good at time management.

For those of you who work in more densely populated cities, getting lunch within walking distance from work is probably a daily routine for you. Instead of ordering delivery, you can order ahead to save time, then speed walk to pick up your food to burn some calories.

Try to do 5-10 minutes of speed walking after you have lunch at work, especially if you know that you will be spending the next few hours sitting in meetings.

Hack #32: Speed walk as much as you can at work.

Chapter 11: Lose Weight Through Sleeping

Now, you have a lot of tricks in your bag that you can use while you are awake to help you lose weight and become more fit. Let's talk about how sleeping can help you lose weight. This might not sound intuitively obvious, especially since a significant portion of the book talks about staying active in order to lose weight.

One thing we all know for sure is that we cannot eat or drink while we sleep. So, sleeping more can reduce our calorie intake frequency and amount. This does not mean that people should sleep 12 hours a day and have no time for exercise or moderate activities. Many people who sleep under 7 hours or less daily struggle to stay energetic, so they often use food and beverages to energize them.

A study has shown that people who increased their sleep duration were able to reduce their caloric intake by an average of 270 kcal per day. That can translate to roughly 12 kg or 26 lbs of weight loss over three years.

When you are well-rested, your brain can make good judgments on calorie intake. When you feel tired or drowsy during the day, your brain tends to make bad decisions when it comes to food, especially when you see something tasty in front of you.

If you feel drowsy only 1 hour after breakfast, it is a sign that you did not get enough sleep. If you find yourself hungry at 11pm at night, it is a sign that you should go to bed instead of heading to the fridge. It is generally recommended that adults sleep 7 or more hours every day.

How much more sleep we need can vary significantly from one person to another. The increase in sleep duration could mean 30 minutes to one person or 1.5 hours to another person. The quality of your sleep matters just as much.

Hack #33: If you are not getting enough sleep, increase your sleep duration to help you lose weight.

Conclusion

Now you understand some of the fundamental barriers to weight loss. More importantly, you have learned 33 simple, easy, and practical hacks to help you lose and keep weight off. Even if you consistently apply 70% of these hacks, you will see measurable results soon. Of course, the more hacks you apply, the sooner and bigger results you will see. In the short term, these hacks can empower you mentally and physically, making your weight loss and fitness journey easier, enjoyable, and sustainable. In the long term, many of these hacks help you live a healthy lifestyle.

You can feel lighter, more energetic, and more confident as early as week 1. Do not wait; take inspired actions today!

Congratulations on finishing the book! It's a significant achievement, and I hope the journey through the book has offered you valuable insights and practical tips for a healthier lifestyle.

P.S. I want to make this journey as easy as possible for you. This book is available in audiobook format, allowing you to listen to the strategies and hacks while on the go and reminding you to make good choices like a coach.

You can scan the QR code below to get the audiobook format.

Resources

Miami Obgyns. (n.d.). Gaining weight in your 40s: Facts and tips – Miami Center of Excellence | Dr. Randy Fink – Miami OBGYNS. Retrieved November 20, 2023, from https://www.miamiobgyns.com/blog/gaining-weight-in-your-40s-facts-and-tips-mcoe/

St-Onge, M., & Gallagher, D. (2010). Body composition changes with aging: The cause or the result of alterations in metabolic rate and macronutrient oxidation? Nutrition, 26(2), 152–155. Retrieved November 20, 2023, from https://www.ncbi.nlm.nih.gov/pmc/articles/PMC2880224/

The reality of menopause weight gain. (2023, July 8). Mayo Clinic. Retrieved November 20, 2023, from https://www.mayoclinic.org/healthy-lifestyle/womens-health/in-depth/menopause-weight-gain/art-20046058

Belly fat in women: Taking — and keeping — it off. (2023, June 28). Mayo Clinic. Retrieved November 20, 2023, from https://www.mayoclinic.org/healthy-lifestyle/womens-health/in-depth/belly-fat/art-20045809#

Yan, Z., Cai, M., Han, X., Chen, Q., & Lu, H. (2023). The Interaction between age and risk factors for diabetes and prediabetes: A Community-Based Cross-Sectional study. Diabetes, Metabolic Syndrome and Obesity: Targets and Therapy, Volume 16, 85–93. Retrieved November 20, 2023, from https://www.ncbi.nlm.nih.gov/pmc/articles/PMC9843502/#

Connected, S. (2023, September 15). More Exercise Doesn't Always Burn More Calories. Science Connected Magazine. Retrieved November 20, 2023, from https://magazine.scienceconnected.org/2021/03/more-exercise-doesnt-always-burn-more-calories/#

Belluz, J., & Haubursin, C. (2019, January 2). The science is in: exercise won't help you lose much weight. Vox. Retrieved November 20, 2023, from https://www.vox.com/2018/1/3/16845438/exercise-weight-loss-myth-burn-calories

Ashton, A., Ashton, A., & Ashton, A. (2021, October 26). How does stress cause belly fat? My Occ Health - Health Workforce, Healthy Business. Retrieved November 20, 2023, from https://www.myocchealth.co.uk/how-does-stress-cause-belly-fat/#

What is cortisol? (2017, February 5). WebMD. Retrieved November 20, 2023, from https://www.webmd.com/a-to-z-guides/what-is-cortisol

BSc, K. G. (2023, June 20). 6 Health benefits of apple cider vinegar, backed by science. Healthline.   Retrieved   November   20,   2023,   from https://www.healthline.com/nutrition/6-proven-health-benefits-of-apple-cider-vinegar#acetic-acid

McAtee, M. (2015, May 4). 7 Benefits of Starting your Day with Lemon Water - LifeQuest Nursing Center. LifeQuest Nursing Center. Retrieved November 20, 2023, from https://www.lifequestnursinghome.org/2015/04/7-benefits-of-starting-your-day-with-lemon-water/#

BSc, K. G. (2023a, February 2). Carbohydrates: Whole vs. Refined — Here's the Difference.   Healthline.   Retrieved   November   20,   2023,   from https://www.healthline.com/nutrition/good-carbs-bad-carbs#

Rd, A. P. M. (2023, August 25). Is Eating While Standing Up Bad for You? Healthline.   Retrieved   November   20,   2023,   from https://www.healthline.com/nutrition/eating-while-standing-up#help-lose-fat

Caldwell, A. (2022, February 7). Getting more sleep reduces caloric intake, a game changer for weight loss programs. UChicagoMedicine. Retrieved November 20, 2023, from   https://www.uchicagomedicine.org/forefront/research-and-discoveries-articles/getting-more-sleep-reduces-caloric-intake#

Paturel, A. (2014, July 6). Sleep more, weigh less. WebMD. Retrieved November 20, 2023, from https://www.webmd.com/diet/sleep-and-weight-loss

How much sleep do I need? (2022, September 14). Centers for Disease Control and Prevention.   Retrieved   November   20,   2023,   from https://www.cdc.gov/sleep/about_sleep/how_much_sleep.html

Weight Loss Hacks for Women Journal

Stop the Weight Loss Saga!

28-Day Journal | Daily Food, Fitness, and Habit Tracker

to Overcome Cravings, Lose Fat, and

Live a Happy, Healthy Lifestyle

Kate M. Right

Introduction

Why is losing weight so damn hard? As someone endlessly curious and analytical with a background steeped in the tech industry, I've always sought to tackle challenges head-on. This resolve led me on a quest for a viable, sustainable approach to weight loss, prompting a deep dive into various diets, fitness, and wellness methodologies. However, the epiphany came not from working harder but from working smarter.

When I shifted my mindset from fixating on limitations to embracing a solution-focused mindset, a simple yet transformative idea struck me: What if I adopt minor habit changes instead of overhauling my entire lifestyle with unmanageable diets and fitness regimes? What if simplicity, rather than complexity, was the key to ending my weight loss saga?

This shift towards straightforward, scientifically-backed strategies for eating, exercising, and daily routines led to astonishing results. I shed 10 pounds in just three weeks and 30 pounds over two months, all while maintaining this new, lighter me. My success story was not just my own. I shared my strategies with friends, which brought them swift, similar results sans starvation or exhaustive gym sessions. This collective success inspired me to author "Weight Loss Hacks for Women Over 40, available on Amazon—a guide to empowering women on their weight loss journeys.

If you're keen on diving straight into action and achieving results without delving into the intricacies, I've prepared a concise cheat sheet that summarizes key strategies in my book as a quick overview. It offers a straightforward approach to rapid, sustainable, and enjoyable weight loss. The daily planner and tracker give you detailed instructions to follow. You could see tangible results as quickly as in 7 days and more significant results within 28 days. Let's get started!

Weight Loss Cheat Sheet

Daily Mindset Exercises:

- Write down a positive affirmation in the present tense three times

- Read your affirmation out loud three times

- Express gratitude out loud or in your mind

Daily Morning Routine:

- Complete the 1-minute mindset exercises when you first wake up

- Weigh yourself before you eat or drink anything; weigh yourself around the same time each morning

- Before you eat anything in the morning, take apple cider vinegar capsules, which can be purchased on Amazon, with a glass of warm water; follow the quantity guidance on the label. Or you can squeeze a fresh lemon into a glass of warm water

- Then, proceed to a healthy breakfast, as outlined for you each day

Daily Smart Nutrition Choices:

- High in lean proteins - animal and/or plant-based

- Moderate in healthy fats - unsaturated fats

- Low-sugar, natural fruits

- Leafy greens with rich fiber, vitamins, and minerals

- Moderate in unprocessed carbs (whole grains), minimize or low in processed carbs (white bread, white rice, white pasta, etc.)

- Low or minimal intake of processed carbs

- Lower in sodium (e.g., use low-sodium salt, low-sodium soy sauce for cooking)

- Low in added sugar

- Drink plenty of water, avoid beverages with added sugar

- If you drink coffee, replace cream/sugar/milk with plant-based milk

Daily Easy Calorie-Burning Habits:

- Do a 20-30 min cardio workout in the gym if you have a gym membership; must vary resistance (e.g., inclination of a treadmill from 5 to 8 to 10 then down to 5) and speed of the cardio machines you use during the workout OR take a 30-min bristle walk if you don't use the gym OR play a sport for 30 minutes

- Take a 20-30 min walk after dinner; you can walk outside or pace inside your home

- Incorporate any style (including lazy style) of sit-ups or push-ups into your media consumption moments—whether you're watching TV, listening to a podcast, or enjoying music. Take your time, and rest as needed between sets. There's no pressure to hit a specific number; do as many repetitions as you're comfortable with. With your attention on the entertainment, you might find yourself breezing through 30 to 50 reps without feeling like a chore

- If possible, try to stand longer instead of sitting for hours when working on computers (e.g., use an adjustable standing desk)

Daily Night Routine:

- Stop eating after 8 pm for at least 5 days each week
- Complete compiling daily scores in the journal
- Reflect on your scores
- Enjoy your "me time" and express gratitude (you can choose from the example list or create your own)
- Go to bed around the same time and make sure you have at least 7+ hours of sleep daily

Note this cheat sheet is a high-level summary of proven strategies from my best-selling weight loss book. Those who have tried numerous weight loss methods might be skeptical about this cheat sheet: these seem to be common sense, nothing earth-shattering. Remember, my breakthrough epiphany was to cut out all the noises and take a simplistic, practical, and sustainable approach to weight loss. The challenge in today's fast-paced information overload age is that even though we know common sense, we struggle to implement common sense. This cheat sheet might seem a bit daunting for those solely focused on dieting, fasting, or exercise. This cheat sheet presents a comprehensive approach to achieving sustainable weight loss and overall fitness. It is only effective if we act on it. To turn this holistic, strategic, and time-efficient approach into easy, actionable steps, I meticulously designed this 3-in-1 journal, planner, and tracker so you can easily incorporate these habit tweaks into your daily life while enjoying this journey.

How to Use This Journal, Planner, and Tracker

This journal, pre-populated with daily weight loss tips, is a step-by-step planner and tracker to guide you in creating mini habits and lasting routines for a healthier lifestyle. Your role in this journey is simple and easy:

1. Each morning, dedicate 1 minute to start your day with a positive mindset. Jot down a positive affirmation three times. Keep the affirmation statement simple and straight to the point. Then, read your affirmation out loud three times and express gratitude. This simple act of repetition is powerful. Feel free to select from the affirmations and gratitude statements provided within or craft your personalized ones.

2. Follow a curated list of actionable steps that span from morning to night and are designed to seamlessly integrate into your daily life.

3. For every action you complete, award yourself one point. At the end of the day, tally your points by category to evaluate your progress. Honesty is essential here—no cheating!

4. At the end of each week, use the reflection page to summarize the past week's experiences and gather insights to enhance your approach for the week ahead.

As mentioned in the introduction, my weight loss strategy is not about overhauling your entire lifestyle suddenly but making incremental habit changes. Hence, you feel in control of your life and enjoy this journey instead of following rigid cooking recipes or exercise routines that you cannot sustain.

You can personalize your calorie-burning habits by increasing the variety of exercise machines or types of activities. The suggested types of activities are intended to make it easy for you to get into the habit of moving your body throughout the day. You can personalize your food choices as long as you eat from the listed nutrition categories daily, which give you quality nutrients and help you feel energetic and full while lowering your overall calorie intake.

With this structured yet flexible system, you'll witness your weight dropping and find joy in the journey towards a healthier you.

Results may vary depending on your metabolic rate before you start this 28-day journey and how closely you follow the step-by-step instructions daily. You will see results even if you apply a fraction of the tips and track your daily progress. Continue to use the journal until you reach your desired weight and fitness goals. But I also recommend that you revisit the journal as often as possible as your health and fitness companion until these healthy habits become your daily routine without thinking about them.

28 Motivational Affirmation Examples

1. I am nourishing my body with healthy foods today.

2. I am so happy that I am losing ___ pounds.

3. I am getting leaner today.

4. I am feeling energetic and stronger.

5. I am reaching my weight loss goal.

6. Every step I take brings me closer to my ideal weight.

7. I am worthy of a healthy and happy life.

8. I celebrate every bit of progress I make.

9. I am becoming a healthier version of myself.

10. My body is a temple, and I treat it with respect.

11. I enjoy the feeling of being fit and energetic.

12. I am in control of my eating habits.

13. I love and accept my body as it transforms.

14. I find joy in physical activity and movement.

15. I am dedicated to improving my health every day

16. I embrace change and welcome new healthy habits.

17. I am proud of myself for every healthy choice I make.

18. I am losing fat and gaining energy.

19. I release all negative thoughts about my body.

20. I am in control of my weight loss journey.

21. My weight loss journey inspires others.

22. I am patient with my body as it changes.

23. I look fabulous, and I love my body.

24. I am achieving a sustainable healthy lifestyle.

25. I deserve to feel good in my body.

26. Weight loss is easy for me.

27. Every day, I grow more energetic and vibrant.

28. I am committed to being the healthiest version of myself.

28 Daily Gratitude Statement Examples

1. I am grateful for my body's ability to move and exercise.

2. I appreciate having healthier food choices.

3. I'm thankful for my energy level today.

4. I am grateful for the strength I gain with each workout.

5. I am so grateful for losing __ pounds.

6. I am thankful for my renewed energy level.

7. Gratitude fills me as I see positive changes in my body.

8. I am thankful for progressing towards my weight loss goal.

9. I am grateful for living a healthier lifestyle.

10. I appreciate my body's resilience and ability to adapt.

11. I am thankful for my sustainable fitness journey.

12. I am grateful for my improved daily routines.

13. I am grateful for the fresh foods that nourish and energize my body.

14. I cherish the moments of rest that rejuvenate my body and mind.

15. I am grateful for this journal that guides me on this 28-day journey.

16. I appreciate the power of positive thinking.

17. I am grateful for my ability to set and achieve my health objectives.

18. I am thankful for the joy that comes from feeling healthier.

19. I am grateful for the discipline I'm developing through.

20. I appreciate every challenge that makes me stronger and more determined.

21. I am thankful for feeling energetic.

22. I am grateful for the lessons learned from setbacks and successes.

23. I am grateful for the peace of mind that comes with a healthy lifestyle.

24. I cherish the journey towards a healthier, happier me.

25. I am thankful for like-minded individuals who inspire me.

26. I appreciate the feeling of vitality that comes with eating well.

27. I am grateful for my smaller waistline.

28. I am thankful for inspiring others with my progress.

Week 1

Date: _____

Day 1

Give 1 point for each item and add total points for each category

Morning Ritual

Upon waking up, start your day with 1-minute positive mental conditioning exercises

MR1. Write down your affirmation in the present tense 3 times

_____

_____

_____   _____

MR2. Read your affirmation out loud in front a mirror and try to feel excited   _____

MR3. Express gratitude mentally or out loud 3 times. It can be as simple as "Thank you" or "I'm grateful for losing weight"   _____

1 point - good start. 2 points - awesome! 3 points excellent!   **Total**   **_____**

Morning - Healthy Eating Habits

M1. Before you eat or drink, record your weight here _____ lbs   _____

M2. Kickstart your metabolism, regulate your blood sugar, curb cravings - drink 8oz of warm water with
   a). Apple cider vinegar capsules OR
   b). Hand squeezed lemon juice   _____

M3. High-nutrient, low-carb breakfast. Include:

1. Lean protein (eggs, smoked salmon, plant-based protein, etc.)   _____
2. Healthy fats (nuts, nut butter, seeds, avocado)   _____
3. Low-sugar raw fruit (orange, berries, melons, apple)   _____
4. Minimally processed carbs, high in fiber (whole grain/wheat)   _____
Optional: Low-sugar, low fat plant-based milk (almond)   _____
3-4 points - good start. 5-6 points - amazing! 7 points - super!   **Total**   **_____**

Lunch - Healthy Eating Habits

L1. High-nutrient, low-carb lunch salads 5 times each week to fuel your body and curb cravings. Include:

1. Lean proteins (eggs, chicken, beef, fish, tofu, etc.) PLUS

2. Leafy greens (arugula, mixed greens) PLUS

3. Your favorite vinegarette dressing (apple, strawberry)

Optional: Low-sugar fruit (orange, berries, avocado, tomatoes)

Optional: Nuts / seeds

Optional - You drink low-sodium, low-carb soup (chick broth, miso soup) to help you feel fuller

Afternoon - Healthy Snacking Habits

A1. Drink 8 oz of water before snacking to curb cravings

A2. High-nutrient, low calorie snacks – total calorie <300

Optional If you drink non-water beverages, there's no added sugar (For coffee/tea, replace sugar/milk/cream with plant-based milk)

4 points - good start. 5-6 points - amazing!

7+ points - you are unstoppable in beating weight gain! **Total**

Dinner - Healthy Eating Habits

D1. High-nutrient, low-carb dinner 5 times each week to fuel your body and curb cravings. Include:

1. Lean proteins (eggs, chicken, beef, fish, tofu, etc.) PLUS

2. Veggies rich in fiber, minerals, vitamins (green beans, spinach, celery, carrot, bok choy, etc.)

3. Minimally processed carbs (brown rice, whole grains)

Optional - Fresh fruit as desert

Bonus: No carbs or consume 50% less carbs than before

Bonus: Only use low-sodium salt / soy sauce for flavor

D2. No eating or snacking after 8pm your time

3 points - good start. 4-5 points - awesome! 6-7 points - excellent! **Total**

WEEK 1

Easy Calorie-Burning Habits
CB1. Worked out for 20-30 min and burned 200+ calories
You applied following techniques to prevent your metabolism from plateauing
a). Used more than 1 type of exercise machine   _____
b). Varied resistance and/or speed of the machine you used   _____
CB2. Instead of going to the gym, you did a 30-min brisk walk or 20-min run or 20-min bike ride   _____
CB3. Did a 30-min sport   _____
CB4. Drank plenty of water after your exercise   _____
CB5. Walked at a moderate speed for 10+ min after lunch   _____
CB6. Took the stairs, skipped the elevator   _____
CB7. Walked at a moderate speed for 20+ min after dinner   _____
Bonus: Did 50 sit-ups and/or 20 push-ups (any style, lazy style) while consuming digital content (e.g., listening to music, pod cast, watching TV) at home   _____
Bonus: If you have an adjustable desk at home or work, you stood while worked at your desk for 60+ minutes   _____
5 – 6 points - good start. 7 – 8 points – amazing!
9+ points - you are on fire!   **Total** _____

Night Time Healthy Habits and Sleep Hygiene
S1. Bedtime - No food past 3 hours & only drank water past 2 hours   _____
S2. Did a calming routine (e.g., meditation, warm bath, journaling, stating affirmations, expressing gratitude, etc.)   _____
S3. Your bed area is device free (your cell phone, tablets, laptops are 5+ feet away and are all turned off)   _____
S4. Your room is noise free and dark once lights are off   _____
S5. Going to bed early to ensure at least 7 hours of sleep   _____
S6. Going to bed around the same time as previous days   _____
S7. Finished tracking points in each category today!   _____
4 points - good start. 5-6 points - great! 7+ points - excellent!   **Total** _____

Notes

_____

_____

_____

_____

_____

_____

_____

_____

Date: _____

Day 2

Give 1 point for each item and add total points for each category

Morning Ritual

Upon waking up, start your day with 1-minute positive mental conditioning exercises

MR1. Write down your affirmation in the present tense 3 times

_____

_____

_____   _____

MR2. Read your affirmation out loud in front a mirror and try to feel excited   _____

MR3. Express gratitude mentally or out loud 3 times. It can be as simple as "Thank you" or "I'm grateful for losing weight"

1 point - good start. 2 points - awesome! 3 points excellent!   **Total**   _____

Morning - Healthy Eating Habits

M1. Before you eat or drink, record your weight here _____ lbs   _____

M2. Kickstart your metabolism, regulate your blood sugar, curb cravings - drink 8oz of warm water with

    a). Apple cider vinegar capsules OR

    b). Hand squeezed lemon juice   _____

M3. High-nutrient, low-carb breakfast. Include:

1. Lean protein (eggs, smoked salmon, plant-based protein, etc.)   _____
2. Healthy fats (nuts, nut butter, seeds, avocado)   _____
3. Low-sugar raw fruit (orange, berries, melons, apple)   _____
4. Minimally processed carbs, high in fiber (whole grain/wheat)   _____

Optional: Low-sugar, low fat plant-based milk (almond)   _____

3-4 points - good start. 5-6 points - amazing! 7 points - super!   **Total**   _____

Lunch - Healthy Eating Habits

L1. High-nutrient, low-carb lunch salads 5 times each week to fuel your body and curb cravings. Include:

1. Lean proteins (eggs, chicken, beef, fish, tofu, etc.) PLUS   _____

2. Leafy greens (arugula, mixed greens) PLUS   _____

3. Your favorite vinegarette dressing (apple, strawberry)   _____

Optional: Low-sugar fruit (orange, berries, avocado, tomatoes)

Optional: Nuts / seeds   _____

Optional - You drink low-sodium, low-carb soup (chick broth, miso soup) to help you feel fuller   _____

Afternoon - Healthy Snacking Habits

A1. Drink 8 oz of water before snacking to curb cravings   _____

A2. High-nutrient, low-calorie snacks – total calorie <300   _____

Optional If you drink non-water beverages, there's no added sugar (For coffee/tea, replace sugar/milk/cream with plant-based milk)   _____

4 points - good start. 5-6 points - amazing!

7+ points - you are unstoppable in beating weight gain!   **Total**   _____

Dinner - Healthy Eating Habits

D1. High-nutrient, low-carb dinner 5 times each week to fuel your body and curb cravings. Include:

1. Lean proteins (eggs, chicken, beef, fish, tofu, etc.) PLUS   _____

2. Veggies rich in fiber, minerals, vitamins (green beans, spinach, celery, carrot, bok choy, etc.)   _____

3. Minimally processed carbs (brown rice, whole grains)   _____

Optional - Fresh fruit as desert   _____

Bonus: No carbs or consume 50% less carbs than before   _____

Bonus: Only use low-sodium salt / soy sauce for flavor   _____

D2. No eating or snacking after 8pm your time   _____

3 points - good start. 4-5 points - awesome! 6-7 points - excellent!   **Total**   _____

Easy Calorie-Burning Habits

CB1. Worked out for 20-30 min and burned 200+ calories
You applied following techniques to prevent your metabolism from plateauing

a). Used more than 1 type of exercise machine _____

b). Varied resistance and/or speed of the machine you used _____

CB2. Instead of going to the gym, you did a 30-min brisk walk or 20-min run or 20-min bike ride _____

CB3. Did a 30-min sport _____

CB4. Drank plenty of water after your exercise _____

CB5. Walked at a moderate speed for 10+ min after lunch _____

CB6. Took the stairs, skipped the elevator _____

CB7. Walked at a moderate speed for 20+ min after dinner _____

Bonus: Did 50 sit-ups and/or 20 push-ups (any style, lazy style) while consuming digital content (e.g., listening to music, pod cast, watching TV) at home _____

Bonus: If you have an adjustable desk at home or work, you stood while worked at your desk for 60+ minutes _____

5 – 6 points - good start. 7 – 8 points – amazing!
9+ points - you are on fire!   **Total** _____

Night Time Healthy Habits and Sleep Hygiene

S1. Bedtime - No food past 3 hours & only drank water past 2 hours _____

S2. Did a calming routine (e.g., meditation, warm bath, journaling, stating affirmations, expressing gratitude, etc.) _____

S3. Your bed area is device free (your cell phone, tablets, laptops are 5+ feet away and are all turned off) _____

S4. Your room is noise free and dark once lights are off _____

S5. Going to bed early to ensure at least 7 hours of sleep _____

S6. Going to bed around the same time as previous days _____

S7. Finished tracking points in each category today! _____

4 points - good start. 5-6 points - great! 7+ points - excellent!   **Total** _____

Notes

_____

_____

_____

_____

_____

_____

_____

_____

Date: _____

Day 3

Give 1 point for each item and add total points for each category

Morning Ritual

Upon waking up, start your day with 1-minute positive mental conditioning exercises

MR1. Write down your affirmation in the present tense 3 times

_____

_____

_____   _____

MR2. Read your affirmation out loud in front a mirror and try to feel excited   _____

MR3. Express gratitude mentally or out loud 3 times. It can be as simple as "Thank you" or "I'm grateful for losing weight"   _____

1 point - good start. 2 points - awesome! 3 points excellent!   **Total**   _____

Morning - Healthy Eating Habits

M1. Before you eat or drink, record your weight here _____ lbs   _____

M2. Kickstart your metabolism, regulate your blood sugar, curb cravings - drink 8oz of warm water with

    a). Apple cider vinegar capsules OR

    b). Hand squeezed lemon juice   _____

M3. High-nutrient, low-carb breakfast. Include:

1. Lean protein (eggs, smoked salmon, plant-based protein, etc.)   _____
2. Healthy fats (nuts, nut butter, seeds, avocado)   _____
3. Low-sugar raw fruit (orange, berries, melons, apple)   _____
4. Minimally processed carbs, high in fiber (whole grain/wheat)   _____

Optional: Low-sugar, low fat plant-based milk (almond)   _____

3-4 points - good start. 5-6 points - amazing! 7 points - super!   **Total**   _____

Lunch - Healthy Eating Habits

L1. High-nutrient, low-carb lunch salads 5 times each week to fuel your body and curb cravings. Include:

1. Lean proteins (eggs, chicken, beef, fish, tofu, etc.) PLUS   _____

2. Leafy greens (arugula, mixed greens) PLUS   _____

3. Your favorite vinegarette dressing (apple, strawberry)   _____

Optional: Low-sugar fruit (orange, berries, avocado, tomatoes)   _____

Optional: Nuts / seeds   _____

Optional - You drink low-sodium, low-carb soup (chick broth, miso soup) to help you feel fuller   _____

Afternoon - Healthy Snacking Habits

A1. Drink 8 oz of water before snacking to curb cravings   _____

A2. High-nutrient, low-calorie snacks – total calorie <300   _____

Optional If you drink non-water beverages, there's no added sugar (For coffee/tea, replace sugar/milk/cream with plant-based milk)   _____

4 points - good start. 5-6 points - amazing!

7+ points - you are unstoppable in beating weight gain!   **Total** _____

Dinner - Healthy Eating Habits

D1. High-nutrient, low-carb dinner 5 times each week to fuel your body and curb cravings. Include:

1. Lean proteins (eggs, chicken, beef, fish, tofu, etc.) PLUS   _____

2. Veggies rich in fiber, minerals, vitamins (green beans, spinach, celery, carrot, bok choy, etc.)   _____

3. Minimally processed carbs (brown rice, whole grains)   _____

Optional - Fresh fruit as desert   _____

Bonus: No carbs or consume 50% less carbs than before   _____

Bonus: Only use low-sodium salt / soy sauce for flavor

D2. No eating or snacking after 8pm your time   _____

3 points - good start. 4-5 points - awesome! 6-7 points - excellent!   **Total** _____

Easy Calorie-Burning Habits
CB1. Worked out for 20-30 min and burned 200+ calories
You applied following techniques to prevent your metabolism from plateauing
a). Used more than 1 type of exercise machine _____
b). Varied resistance and/or speed of the machine you used _____
CB2. Instead of going to the gym, you did a 30-min brisk walk or 20-min run or 20-min bike ride _____
CB3. Did a 30-min sport _____
CB4. Drank plenty of water after your exercise _____
CB5. Walked at a moderate speed for 10+ min after lunch _____
CB6. Took the stairs, skipped the elevator _____
CB7. Walked at a moderate speed for 20+ min after dinner _____
Bonus: Did 50 sit-ups and/or 20 push-ups (any style, lazy style) while consuming digital content (e.g., listening to music, pod cast, watching TV) at home _____
Bonus: If you have an adjustable desk at home or work, you stood while worked at your desk for 60+ minutes _____
5 – 6 points - good start. 7 – 8 points – amazing!
9+ points - you are on fire!   **Total** _____

Night Time Healthy Habits and Sleep Hygiene
S1. Bedtime - No food past 3 hours & only drank water past 2 hours _____
S2. Did a calming routine (e.g., meditation, warm bath, journaling, stating affirmations, expressing gratitude, etc.) _____
S3. Your bed area is device free (your cell phone, tablets, laptops are 5+ feet away and are all turned off) _____
S4. Your room is noise free and dark once lights are off _____
S5. Going to bed early to ensure at least 7 hours of sleep _____
S6. Going to bed around the same time as previous days _____
S7. Finished tracking points in each category today! _____
4 points - good start. 5-6 points - great! 7+ points - excellent!   **Total** _____

Notes

_____

_____

_____

_____

_____

_____

_____

_____

Date: _____

Day 4

Give 1 point for each item and add total points for each category

Morning Ritual

Upon waking up, start your day with 1-minute positive mental conditioning exercises

MR1. Write down your affirmation in the present tense 3 times

_____

_____

_____ _____

MR2. Read your affirmation out loud in front a mirror and try to feel excited _____

MR3. Express gratitude mentally or out loud 3 times. It can be as simple as "Thank you" or "I'm grateful for losing weight" _____

1 point - good start. 2 points - awesome! 3 points excellent! **Total** _____

Morning - Healthy Eating Habits

M1. Before you eat or drink, record your weight here _____ lbs _____

M2. Kickstart your metabolism, regulate your blood sugar, curb cravings - drink 8oz of warm water with

   a). Apple cider vinegar capsules OR

   b). Hand squeezed lemon juice _____

M3. High-nutrient, low-carb breakfast. Include:

1. Lean protein (eggs, smoked salmon, plant-based protein, etc.) _____
2. Healthy fats (nuts, nut butter, seeds, avocado) _____
3. Low-sugar raw fruit (orange, berries, melons, apple) _____
4. Minimally processed carbs, high in fiber (whole grain/wheat) _____
Optional: Low-sugar, low fat plant-based milk (almond) _____

3-4 points - good start. 5-6 points - amazing! 7 points - super! **Total** _____

Lunch - Healthy Eating Habits

L1. High-nutrient, low-carb lunch salads 5 times each week to fuel your body and curb cravings. Include:

1. Lean proteins (eggs, chicken, beef, fish, tofu, etc.) PLUS _____

2. Leafy greens (arugula, mixed greens) PLUS _____

3. Your favorite vinegarette dressing (apple, strawberry) _____

Optional: Low-sugar fruit (orange, berries, avocado, tomatoes) _____

Optional: Nuts / seeds _____

Optional - You drink low-sodium, low-carb soup (chick broth, miso soup) to help you feel fuller _____

Afternoon - Healthy Snacking Habits

A1. Drink 8 oz of water before snacking to curb cravings _____

A2. High-nutrient, low-calorie snacks – total calorie <300 _____

Optional If you drink non-water beverages, there's no added sugar (For coffee/tea, replace sugar/milk/cream with plant-based milk) _____

4 points - good start. 5-6 points - amazing!

7+ points - you are unstoppable in beating weight gain!   **Total** _____

Dinner - Healthy Eating Habits

D1. High-nutrient, low-carb dinner 5 times each week to fuel your body and curb cravings. Include:

1. Lean proteins (eggs, chicken, beef, fish, tofu, etc.) PLUS _____

2. Veggies rich in fiber, minerals, vitamins (green beans, spinach, celery, carrot, bok choy, etc.) _____

3. Minimally processed carbs (brown rice, whole grains) _____

Optional - Fresh fruit as desert _____

Bonus: No carbs or consume 50% less carbs than before _____

Bonus: Only use low-sodium salt / soy sauce for flavor _____

D2. No eating or snacking after 8pm your time _____

3 points - good start. 4-5 points - awesome! 6-7 points - excellent!   **Total** _____

Easy Calorie-Burning Habits

CB1. Worked out for 20-30 min and burned 200+ calories

You applied following techniques to prevent your metabolism from plateauing

a). Used more than 1 type of exercise machine   _____

b). Varied resistance and/or speed of the machine you used   _____

CB2. Instead of going to the gym, you did a 30-min brisk walk or 20-min run or 20-min bike ride   _____

CB3. Did a 30-min sport   _____

CB4. Drank plenty of water after your exercise   _____

CB5. Walked at a moderate speed for 10+ min after lunch   _____

CB6. Took the stairs, skipped the elevator   _____

CB7. Walked at a moderate speed for 20+ min after dinner   _____

Bonus: Did 50 sit-ups and/or 20 push-ups (any style, lazy style) while consuming digital content (e.g., listening to music, pod cast, watching TV) at home   _____

Bonus: If you have an adjustable desk at home or work, you stood while worked at your desk for 60+ minutes   _____

5 – 6 points - good start. 7 – 8 points – amazing!

9+ points - you are on fire!   **Total** _____

Night Time Healthy Habits and Sleep Hygiene

S1. Bedtime - No food past 3 hours & only drank water past 2 hours   _____

S2. Did a calming routine (e.g., meditation, warm bath, journaling, stating affirmations, expressing gratitude, etc.)   _____

S3. Your bed area is device free (your cell phone, tablets, laptops are 5+ feet away and are all turned off)   _____

S4. Your room is noise free and dark once lights are off   _____

S5. Going to bed early to ensure at least 7 hours of sleep   _____

S6. Going to bed around the same time as previous days   _____

S7. Finished tracking points in each category today!   _____

4 points - good start. 5-6 points - great! 7+ points - excellent!   **Total** _____

Notes

Date: _____

Day 5

Give 1 point for each item and add total points for each category

Morning Ritual

Upon waking up, start your day with 1-minute positive mental conditioning exercises

MR1. Write down your affirmation in the present tense 3 times

_____

_____

_____ _____

MR2. Read your affirmation out loud in front a mirror and try to feel excited _____

MR3. Express gratitude mentally or out loud 3 times. It can be as simple as "Thank you" or "I'm grateful for losing weight" _____

1 point - good start. 2 points - awesome! 3 points excellent! **Total** _____

Morning - Healthy Eating Habits

M1. Before you eat or drink, record your weight here _____ lbs _____

M2. Kickstart your metabolism, regulate your blood sugar, curb cravings - drink 8oz of warm water with

    a). Apple cider vinegar capsules OR

    b). Hand squeezed lemon juice _____

M3. High-nutrient, low-carb breakfast. Include:

1. Lean protein (eggs, smoked salmon, plant-based protein, etc.) _____
2. Healthy fats (nuts, nut butter, seeds, avocado) _____
3. Low-sugar raw fruit (orange, berries, melons, apple) _____
4. Minimally processed carbs, high in fiber (whole grain/wheat) _____

Optional: Low-sugar, low fat plant-based milk (almond) _____

3-4 points - good start. 5-6 points - amazing! 7 points - super! **Total** _____

Lunch - Healthy Eating Habits

L1. High-nutrient, low-carb lunch salads 5 times each week to fuel your body and curb cravings. Include:

1. Lean proteins (eggs, chicken, beef, fish, tofu, etc.) PLUS   _____

2. Leafy greens (arugula, mixed greens) PLUS   _____

3. Your favorite vinegarette dressing (apple, strawberry)   _____

Optional: Low-sugar fruit (orange, berries, avocado, tomatoes)   _____

Optional: Nuts / seeds   _____

Optional - You drink low-sodium, low-carb soup (chick broth, miso soup) to help you feel fuller   _____

Afternoon - Healthy Snacking Habits

A1. Drink 8 oz of water before snacking to curb cravings   _____

A2. High-nutrient, low-calorie snacks – total calorie <300   _____

Optional If you drink non-water beverages, there's no added sugar (For coffee/tea, replace sugar/milk/cream with plant-based milk)   _____

4 points - good start. 5-6 points - amazing!

7+ points - you are unstoppable in beating weight gain!   **Total** _____

Dinner - Healthy Eating Habits

D1. High-nutrient, low-carb dinner 5 times each week to fuel your body and curb cravings. Include:

1. Lean proteins (eggs, chicken, beef, fish, tofu, etc.) PLUS   _____

2. Veggies rich in fiber, minerals, vitamins (green beans, spinach, celery, carrot, bok choy, etc.)   _____

3. Minimally processed carbs (brown rice, whole grains)   _____

Optional - Fresh fruit as desert   _____

Bonus: No carbs or consume 50% less carbs than before   _____

Bonus: Only use low-sodium salt / soy sauce for flavor   _____

D2. No eating or snacking after 8pm your time   _____

3 points - good start. 4-5 points - awesome! 6-7 points - excellent!   **Total** _____

Easy Calorie-Burning Habits

CB1. Worked out for 20-30 min and burned 200+ calories

You applied following techniques to prevent your metabolism from plateauing

a). Used more than 1 type of exercise machine _____

b). Varied resistance and/or speed of the machine you used _____

CB2. Instead of going to the gym, you did a 30-min brisk walk or 20-min run or 20-min bike ride _____

CB3. Did a 30-min sport _____

CB4. Drank plenty of water after your exercise _____

CB5. Walked at a moderate speed for 10+ min after lunch _____

CB6. Took the stairs, skipped the elevator _____

CB7. Walked at a moderate speed for 20+ min after dinner _____

Bonus: Did 50 sit-ups and/or 20 push-ups (any style, lazy style) while consuming digital content (e.g., listening to music, pod cast, watching TV) at home _____

Bonus: If you have an adjustable desk at home or work, you stood while worked at your desk for 60+ minutes _____

5 – 6 points - good start. 7 – 8 points – amazing!

9+ points - you are on fire!   **Total** _____

Night Time Healthy Habits and Sleep Hygiene

S1. Bedtime - No food past 3 hours & only drank water past 2 hours _____

S2. Did a calming routine (e.g., meditation, warm bath, journaling, stating affirmations, expressing gratitude, etc.) _____

S3. Your bed area is device free (your cell phone, tablets, laptops are 5+ feet away and are all turned off) _____

S4. Your room is noise free and dark once lights are off _____

S5. Going to bed early to ensure at least 7 hours of sleep _____

S6. Going to bed around the same time as previous days _____

S7. Finished tracking points in each category today! _____

4 points - good start. 5-6 points - great! 7+ points - excellent!   **Total** _____

Notes

Date: _____

Day 6

Give 1 point for each item and add total points for each category

Morning Ritual

Upon waking up, start your day with 1-minute positive mental conditioning exercises

MR1. Write down your affirmation in the present tense 3 times

_____

_____

_____   _____

MR2. Read your affirmation out loud in front a mirror and try to feel excited   _____

MR3. Express gratitude mentally or out loud 3 times. It can be as simple as "Thank you" or "I'm grateful for losing weight"   _____

1 point - good start. 2 points - awesome! 3 points excellent!   **Total** _____

Morning - Healthy Eating Habits

M1. Before you eat or drink, record your weight here _____ lbs   _____

M2. Kickstart your metabolism, regulate your blood sugar, curb cravings - drink 8oz of warm water with

   a). Apple cider vinegar capsules OR

   b). Hand squeezed lemon juice   _____

M3. High-nutrient, low-carb breakfast. Include:

1. Lean protein (eggs, smoked salmon, plant-based protein, etc.)   _____
2. Healthy fats (nuts, nut butter, seeds, avocado)   _____
3. Low-sugar raw fruit (orange, berries, melons, apple)   _____
4. Minimally processed carbs, high in fiber (whole grain/wheat)   _____

Optional: Low-sugar, low fat plant-based milk (almond)   _____

3-4 points - good start. 5-6 points - amazing! 7 points - super!   **Total** _____

Lunch - Healthy Eating Habits

L1. High-nutrient, low-carb lunch salads 5 times each week to fuel your body and curb cravings. Include:

1. Lean proteins (eggs, chicken, beef, fish, tofu, etc.) PLUS _____

2. Leafy greens (arugula, mixed greens) PLUS _____

3. Your favorite vinegarette dressing (apple, strawberry) _____

Optional: Low-sugar fruit (orange, berries, avocado, tomatoes)

Optional: Nuts / seeds _____

Optional - You drink low-sodium, low-carb soup (chick broth, miso soup) to help you feel fuller _____

Afternoon - Healthy Snacking Habits

A1. Drink 8 oz of water before snacking to curb cravings _____

A2. High-nutrient, low-calorie snacks – total calorie <300 _____

Optional If you drink non-water beverages, there's no added sugar (For coffee/tea, replace sugar/milk/cream with plant-based milk) _____

4 points - good start. 5-6 points - amazing!

7+ points - you are unstoppable in beating weight gain! **Total** _____

Dinner - Healthy Eating Habits

D1. High-nutrient, low-carb dinner 5 times each week to fuel your body and curb cravings. Include:

1. Lean proteins (eggs, chicken, beef, fish, tofu, etc.) PLUS _____

2. Veggies rich in fiber, minerals, vitamins (green beans, spinach, celery, carrot, bok choy, etc.) _____

3. Minimally processed carbs (brown rice, whole grains) _____

Optional - Fresh fruit as desert _____

Bonus: No carbs or consume 50% less carbs than before _____

Bonus: Only use low-sodium salt / soy sauce for flavor _____

D2. No eating or snacking after 8pm your time _____

3 points - good start. 4-5 points - awesome! 6-7 points - excellent! **Total** _____

Easy Calorie-Burning Habits
CB1. Worked out for 20-30 min and burned 200+ calories
You applied following techniques to prevent your metabolism from plateauing
a). Used more than 1 type of exercise machine _____
b). Varied resistance and/or speed of the machine you used _____
CB2. Instead of going to the gym, you did a 30-min brisk walk or 20-min run or 20-min bike ride _____
CB3. Did a 30-min sport _____
CB4. Drank plenty of water after your exercise _____
CB5. Walked at a moderate speed for 10+ min after lunch _____
CB6. Took the stairs, skipped the elevator _____
CB7. Walked at a moderate speed for 20+ min after dinner _____
Bonus: Did 50 sit-ups and/or 20 push-ups (any style, lazy style) while consuming digital content (e.g., listening to music, pod cast, watching TV) at home _____
Bonus: If you have an adjustable desk at home or work, you stood while worked at your desk for 60+ minutes _____
5 – 6 points - good start. 7 – 8 points – amazing!
9+ points - you are on fire! **Total** _____

Night Time Healthy Habits and Sleep Hygiene
S1. Bedtime - No food past 3 hours & only drank water past 2 hours _____
S2. Did a calming routine (e.g., meditation, warm bath, journaling, stating affirmations, expressing gratitude, etc.) _____
S3. Your bed area is device free (your cell phone, tablets, laptops are 5+ feet away and are all turned off) _____
S4. Your room is noise free and dark once lights are off _____
S5. Going to bed early to ensure at least 7 hours of sleep _____
S6. Going to bed around the same time as previous days _____
S7. Finished tracking points in each category today! _____
4 points - good start. 5-6 points - great! 7+ points - excellent! **Total** _____

Notes

_____

_____

_____

_____

_____

_____

_____

_____

Date: _____

Day 7

Give 1 point for each item and add total points for each category

Morning Ritual

Upon waking up, start your day with 1-minute positive mental conditioning exercises

MR1. Write down your affirmation in the present tense 3 times

_____

_____

_____   _____

MR2. Read your affirmation out loud in front a mirror and try to feel excited   _____

MR3. Express gratitude mentally or out loud 3 times. It can be as simple as "Thank you" or "I'm grateful for losing weight"   _____

1 point - good start. 2 points - awesome! 3 points excellent!   **Total**   _____

Morning - Healthy Eating Habits

M1. Before you eat or drink, record your weight here _____ lbs   _____

M2. Kickstart your metabolism, regulate your blood sugar, curb cravings - drink 8oz of warm water with

   a). Apple cider vinegar capsules OR

   b). Hand squeezed lemon juice   _____

M3. High-nutrient, low-carb breakfast. Include:

1. Lean protein (eggs, smoked salmon, plant-based protein, etc.)   _____
2. Healthy fats (nuts, nut butter, seeds, avocado)   _____
3. Low-sugar raw fruit (orange, berries, melons, apple)   _____
4. Minimally processed carbs, high in fiber (whole grain/wheat)   _____

Optional: Low-sugar, low fat plant-based milk (almond)   _____

3-4 points - good start. 5-6 points - amazing! 7 points - super!   **Total**   _____

Lunch - Healthy Eating Habits

L1. High-nutrient, low-carb lunch salads 5 times each week to fuel your body and curb cravings. Include:

1. Lean proteins (eggs, chicken, beef, fish, tofu, etc.) PLUS _____

2. Leafy greens (arugula, mixed greens) PLUS _____

3. Your favorite vinegarette dressing (apple, strawberry) _____

Optional: Low-sugar fruit (orange, berries, avocado, tomatoes) _____

Optional: Nuts / seeds _____

Optional - You drink low-sodium, low-carb soup (chick broth, miso soup) to help you feel fuller _____

Afternoon - Healthy Snacking Habits

A1. Drink 8 oz of water before snacking to curb cravings _____

A2. High-nutrient, low-calorie snacks – total calorie <300 _____

Optional If you drink non-water beverages, there's no added sugar (For coffee/tea, replace sugar/milk/cream with plant-based milk) _____

4 points - good start. 5-6 points - amazing!

7+ points - you are unstoppable in beating weight gain! **Total** _____

Dinner - Healthy Eating Habits

D1. High-nutrient, low-carb dinner 5 times each week to fuel your body and curb cravings. Include:

1. Lean proteins (eggs, chicken, beef, fish, tofu, etc.) PLUS _____

2. Veggies rich in fiber, minerals, vitamins (green beans, spinach, celery, carrot, bok choy, etc.) _____

3. Minimally processed carbs (brown rice, whole grains) _____

Optional - Fresh fruit as desert _____

Bonus: No carbs or consume 50% less carbs than before

Bonus: Only use low-sodium salt / soy sauce for flavor

D2. No eating or snacking after 8pm your time _____

3 points - good start. 4-5 points - awesome! 6-7 points - excellent! **Total** _____

Easy Calorie-Burning Habits
CB1. Worked out for 20-30 min and burned 200+ calories
You applied following techniques to prevent your metabolism from plateauing
a). Used more than 1 type of exercise machine   _____
b). Varied resistance and/or speed of the machine you used   _____
CB2. Instead of going to the gym, you did a 30-min brisk walk or 20-min run or 20-min bike ride   _____
CB3. Did a 30-min sport   _____
CB4. Drank plenty of water after your exercise   _____
CB5. Walked at a moderate speed for 10+ min after lunch   _____
CB6. Took the stairs, skipped the elevator   _____
CB7. Walked at a moderate speed for 20+ min after dinner   _____
Bonus: Did 50 sit-ups and/or 20 push-ups (any style, lazy style) while consuming digital content (e.g., listening to music, pod cast, watching TV) at home   _____
Bonus: If you have an adjustable desk at home or work, you stood while worked at your desk for 60+ minutes   _____
5 – 6 points - good start. 7 – 8 points – amazing!
9+ points - you are on fire!   **Total** _____

Night Time Healthy Habits and Sleep Hygiene
S1. Bedtime - No food past 3 hours & only drank water past 2 hours   _____
S2. Did a calming routine (e.g., meditation, warm bath, journaling, stating affirmations, expressing gratitude, etc.)   _____
S3. Your bed area is device free (your cell phone, tablets, laptops are 5+ feet away and are all turned off)   _____
S4. Your room is noise free and dark once lights are off   _____
S5. Going to bed early to ensure at least 7 hours of sleep   _____
S6. Going to bed around the same time as previous days   _____
S7. Finished tracking points in each category today!   _____
4 points - good start. 5-6 points - great! 7+ points - excellent!   **Total** _____

Notes

Date: _____

End of Week 1 Reflection

Day 1 weight _____   Day 7 weight _____

Which habit categories you ...	...consistently scored well?	...consistently scored lower (good start)?	...plan to improve the most next week?
Morning Ritual			
Morning Healthy Eating Habits			
Lunch Healthy Eating + Afternoon Healthy Snacking Habits			
Dinner Healthy Eating Habits			
Calorie-Burning Habits			
Night Time Healthy Habits and Sleep Hygiene			

Pat yourself on the back even if your weight roughly stayed the same this week. The fact that you have completed this entire week's habit tracking is a win! Celebrate every win, small or big. Just don't binge-eat your guilty pleasures. Take everything in moderation and you will see and feel the rewards of living a healthy lifestyle.

If your weight increases, which could very well be water retention caused by menstruation, high-sodium foods, or high-carb foods, continue the daily habits next week. As long as you try to improve the categories you scored low this week, you will see tangible weight loss soon.

State these gratitude statements out loud 3 times and try to feel your weight loss outcomes and get excited:

- I am so grateful for feeling lighter, leaner and more energetic!
- I am so grateful for completing daily habit tracking.
- I am so grateful for putting high-nutrient foods in my body and keeping myself

active.

Week 2

Date: _____

Day 1

Give 1 point for each item and add total points for each category

Morning Ritual

Upon waking up, start your day with 1-minute positive mental conditioning exercises

MR1. Write down your affirmation in the present tense 3 times

_____

_____

_____   _____

MR2. Read your affirmation out loud in front a mirror and try to feel excited   _____

MR3. Express gratitude mentally or out loud 3 times. It can be as simple as "Thank you" or "I'm grateful for losing weight"   _____

1 point - good start. 2 points - awesome! 3 points excellent!   **Total** _____

Morning - Healthy Eating Habits

M1. Before you eat or drink, record your weight here _____ lbs   _____

M2. Kickstart your metabolism, regulate your blood sugar, curb cravings - drink 8oz of warm water with

    a). Apple cider vinegar capsules OR

    b). Hand squeezed lemon juice   _____

M3. High-nutrient, low-carb breakfast. Include:

1. Lean protein (eggs, smoked salmon, plant-based protein, etc.)   _____
2. Healthy fats (nuts, nut butter, seeds, avocado)   _____
3. Low-sugar raw fruit (orange, berries, melons, apple)   _____
4. Minimally processed carbs, high in fiber (whole grain/wheat)   _____
Optional: Low-sugar, low fat plant-based milk (almond)   _____
3-4 points - good start. 5-6 points - amazing! 7 points - super! **Total** _____

Lunch - Healthy Eating Habits
L1. High-nutrient, low-carb lunch salads 5 times each week to fuel your body and curb cravings. Include:
1. Lean proteins (eggs, chicken, beef, fish, tofu, etc.) PLUS   _____
2. Leafy greens (arugula, mixed greens) PLUS   _____
3. Your favorite vinegarette dressing (apple, strawberry)   _____
Optional: Low-sugar fruit (orange, berries, avocado, tomatoes)   _____
Optional: Nuts / seeds   _____
Optional - You drink low-sodium, low-carb soup (chick broth, miso soup) to help you feel fuller   _____

Afternoon - Healthy Snacking Habits
A1. Drink 8 oz of water before snacking to curb cravings   _____
A2. High-nutrient, low-calorie snacks – total calorie <300   _____
Optional If you drink non-water beverages, there's no added sugar (For coffee/tea, replace sugar/milk/cream with plant-based milk)   _____
4 points - good start. 5-6 points - amazing!
7+ points - you are unstoppable in beating weight gain!   **Total** _____

Dinner - Healthy Eating Habits
D1. High-nutrient, low-carb dinner 5 times each week to fuel your body and curb cravings. Include:
1. Lean proteins (eggs, chicken, beef, fish, tofu, etc.) PLUS   _____
2. Veggies rich in fiber, minerals, vitamins (green beans, spinach, celery, carrot, bok choy, etc.)   _____
3. Minimally processed carbs (brown rice, whole grains)   _____
Optional - Fresh fruit as desert   _____
Bonus: No carbs or consume 50% less carbs than before   _____
Bonus: Only use low-sodium salt / soy sauce for flavor   _____
D2. No eating or snacking after 8pm your time   _____
3 points - good start. 4-5 points - awesome! 6-7 points - excellent!   **Total** _____

Easy Calorie-Burning Habits

CB1. Worked out for 20-30 min and burned 200+ calories

You applied following techniques to prevent your metabolism from plateauing

a). Used more than 1 type of exercise machine _____

b). Varied resistance and/or speed of the machine you used _____

CB2. Instead of going to the gym, you did a 30-min brisk walk or 20-min run or 20-min bike ride _____

CB3. Did a 30-min sport _____

CB4. Drank plenty of water after your exercise _____

CB5. Walked at a moderate speed for 10+ min after lunch _____

CB6. Took the stairs, skipped the elevator _____

CB7. Walked at a moderate speed for 20+ min after dinner _____

Bonus: Did 50 sit-ups and/or 20 push-ups (any style, lazy style) while consuming digital content (e.g., listening to music, pod cast, watching TV) at home _____

Bonus: If you have an adjustable desk at home or work, you stood while worked at your desk for 60+ minutes _____

5 – 6 points - good start. 7 – 8 points – amazing!

9+ points - you are on fire!   **Total** _____

Night Time Healthy Habits and Sleep Hygiene

S1. Bedtime - No food past 3 hours & only drank water past 2 hours _____

S2. Did a calming routine (e.g., meditation, warm bath, journaling, stating affirmations, expressing gratitude, etc.) _____

S3. Your bed area is device free (your cell phone, tablets, laptops are 5+ feet away and are all turned off) _____

S4. Your room is noise free and dark once lights are off _____

S5. Going to bed early to ensure at least 7 hours of sleep _____

S6. Going to bed around the same time as previous days _____

S7. Finished tracking points in each category today! _____

4 points - good start. 5-6 points - great! 7+ points - excellent!   **Total** _____

Notes

Date: _____

Day 2

Give 1 point for each item and add total points for each category

Morning Ritual

Upon waking up, start your day with 1-minute positive mental conditioning exercises

MR1. Write down your affirmation in the present tense 3 times

_____

_____

_____   _____

MR2. Read your affirmation out loud in front a mirror and try to feel excited   _____

MR3. Express gratitude mentally or out loud 3 times. It can be as simple as "Thank you" or "I'm grateful for losing weight"   _____

1 point - good start. 2 points - awesome! 3 points excellent!   **Total**   _____

Morning - Healthy Eating Habits

M1. Before you eat or drink, record your weight here _____ lbs   _____

M2. Kickstart your metabolism, regulate your blood sugar, curb cravings - drink 8oz of warm water with

   a). Apple cider vinegar capsules OR

   b). Hand squeezed lemon juice   _____

M3. High-nutrient, low-carb breakfast. Include:

1. Lean protein (eggs, smoked salmon, plant-based protein, etc.)   _____
2. Healthy fats (nuts, nut butter, seeds, avocado)   _____
3. Low-sugar raw fruit (orange, berries, melons, apple)   _____
4. Minimally processed carbs, high in fiber (whole grain/wheat)   _____

Optional: Low-sugar, low fat plant-based milk (almond)   _____

3-4 points - good start. 5-6 points - amazing! 7 points - super!   **Total**   _____

Lunch - Healthy Eating Habits

L1. High-nutrient, low-carb lunch salads 5 times each week to fuel your body and curb cravings. Include:

1. Lean proteins (eggs, chicken, beef, fish, tofu, etc.) PLUS _____

2. Leafy greens (arugula, mixed greens) PLUS _____

3. Your favorite vinegarette dressing (apple, strawberry) _____

Optional: Low-sugar fruit (orange, berries, avocado, tomatoes) _____

Optional: Nuts / seeds _____

Optional - You drink low-sodium, low-carb soup (chick broth, miso soup) to help you feel fuller _____

Afternoon - Healthy Snacking Habits

A1. Drink 8 oz of water before snacking to curb cravings _____

A2. High-nutrient, low-calorie snacks – total calorie <300 _____

Optional If you drink non-water beverages, there's no added sugar (For coffee/tea, replace sugar/milk/cream with plant-based milk) _____

4 points - good start. 5-6 points - amazing!

7+ points - you are unstoppable in beating weight gain! **Total** _____

Dinner - Healthy Eating Habits

D1. High-nutrient, low-carb dinner 5 times each week to fuel your body and curb cravings. Include:

1. Lean proteins (eggs, chicken, beef, fish, tofu, etc.) PLUS _____

2. Veggies rich in fiber, minerals, vitamins (green beans, spinach, celery, carrot, bok choy, etc.) _____

3. Minimally processed carbs (brown rice, whole grains) _____

Optional - Fresh fruit as desert _____

Bonus: No carbs or consume 50% less carbs than before _____

Bonus: Only use low-sodium salt / soy sauce for flavor _____

D2. No eating or snacking after 8pm your time _____

3 points - good start. 4-5 points - awesome! 6-7 points - excellent! **Total** _____

Easy Calorie-Burning Habits

CB1. Worked out for 20-30 min and burned 200+ calories
You applied following techniques to prevent your metabolism from plateauing

a). Used more than 1 type of exercise machine _____

b). Varied resistance and/or speed of the machine you used _____

CB2. Instead of going to the gym, you did a 30-min brisk walk or 20-min run or 20-min bike ride _____

CB3. Did a 30-min sport _____

CB4. Drank plenty of water after your exercise _____

CB5. Walked at a moderate speed for 10+ min after lunch _____

CB6. Took the stairs, skipped the elevator _____

CB7. Walked at a moderate speed for 20+ min after dinner _____

Bonus: Did 50 sit-ups and/or 20 push-ups (any style, lazy style) while consuming digital content (e.g., listening to music, pod cast, watching TV) at home _____

Bonus: If you have an adjustable desk at home or work, you stood while worked at your desk for 60+ minutes _____

5 – 6 points - good start. 7 – 8 points – amazing!
9+ points - you are on fire!   **Total** _____

Night Time Healthy Habits and Sleep Hygiene

S1. Bedtime - No food past 3 hours & only drank water past 2 hours _____

S2. Did a calming routine (e.g., meditation, warm bath, journaling, stating affirmations, expressing gratitude, etc.) _____

S3. Your bed area is device free (your cell phone, tablets, laptops are 5+ feet away and are all turned off) _____

S4. Your room is noise free and dark once lights are off _____

S5. Going to bed early to ensure at least 7 hours of sleep _____

S6. Going to bed around the same time as previous days _____

S7. Finished tracking points in each category today! _____

4 points - good start. 5-6 points - great! 7+ points - excellent!   **Total** _____

Notes

Date: _____

Day 3

Give 1 point for each item and add total points for each category

Morning Ritual

Upon waking up, start your day with 1-minute positive mental conditioning exercises

MR1. Write down your affirmation in the present tense 3 times

_____

_____

_____   _____

MR2. Read your affirmation out loud in front a mirror and try to feel excited   _____

MR3. Express gratitude mentally or out loud 3 times. It can be as simple as "Thank you" or "I'm grateful for losing weight"   _____

1 point - good start. 2 points - awesome! 3 points excellent!   **Total**   _____

Morning - Healthy Eating Habits

M1. Before you eat or drink, record your weight here _____ lbs   _____

M2. Kickstart your metabolism, regulate your blood sugar, curb cravings - drink 8oz of warm water with

   a). Apple cider vinegar capsules OR

   b). Hand squeezed lemon juice   _____

M3. High-nutrient, low-carb breakfast. Include:

1. Lean protein (eggs, smoked salmon, plant-based protein, etc.)   _____
2. Healthy fats (nuts, nut butter, seeds, avocado)   _____
3. Low-sugar raw fruit (orange, berries, melons, apple)   _____
4. Minimally processed carbs, high in fiber (whole grain/wheat)   _____

Optional: Low-sugar, low fat plant-based milk (almond)   _____

3-4 points - good start. 5-6 points - amazing! 7 points - super!   **Total**   _____

Lunch - Healthy Eating Habits

L1. High-nutrient, low-carb lunch salads 5 times each week to fuel your body and curb cravings. Include:

1. Lean proteins (eggs, chicken, beef, fish, tofu, etc.) PLUS _____

2. Leafy greens (arugula, mixed greens) PLUS _____

3. Your favorite vinegarette dressing (apple, strawberry) _____

Optional: Low-sugar fruit (orange, berries, avocado, tomatoes) _____

Optional: Nuts / seeds _____

Optional - You drink low-sodium, low-carb soup (chick broth, miso soup) to help you feel fuller _____

Afternoon - Healthy Snacking Habits

A1. Drink 8 oz of water before snacking to curb cravings _____

A2. High-nutrient, low-calorie snacks – total calorie <300 _____

Optional If you drink non-water beverages, there's no added sugar (For coffee/tea, replace sugar/milk/cream with plant-based milk) _____

4 points - good start. 5-6 points - amazing!

7+ points - you are unstoppable in beating weight gain!   **Total** _____

Dinner - Healthy Eating Habits

D1. High-nutrient, low-carb dinner 5 times each week to fuel your body and curb cravings. Include:

1. Lean proteins (eggs, chicken, beef, fish, tofu, etc.) PLUS _____

2. Veggies rich in fiber, minerals, vitamins (green beans, spinach, celery, carrot, bok choy, etc.) _____

3. Minimally processed carbs (brown rice, whole grains) _____

Optional - Fresh fruit as desert _____

Bonus: No carbs or consume 50% less carbs than before _____

Bonus: Only use low-sodium salt / soy sauce for flavor _____

D2. No eating or snacking after 8pm your time _____

3 points - good start. 4-5 points - awesome! 6-7 points - excellent!   **Total** _____

Easy Calorie-Burning Habits
CB1. Worked out for 20-30 min and burned 200+ calories
You applied following techniques to prevent your metabolism from plateauing
a). Used more than 1 type of exercise machine _____
b). Varied resistance and/or speed of the machine you used _____
CB2. Instead of going to the gym, you did a 30-min brisk walk or 20-min run or 20-min bike ride _____
CB3. Did a 30-min sport _____
CB4. Drank plenty of water after your exercise _____
CB5. Walked at a moderate speed for 10+ min after lunch _____
CB6. Took the stairs, skipped the elevator _____
CB7. Walked at a moderate speed for 20+ min after dinner _____
Bonus: Did 50 sit-ups and/or 20 push-ups (any style, lazy style) while consuming digital content (e.g., listening to music, pod cast, watching TV) at home _____
Bonus: If you have an adjustable desk at home or work, you stood while worked at your desk for 60+ minutes _____
5 – 6 points - good start. 7 – 8 points – amazing!
9+ points - you are on fire! **Total** _____

Night Time Healthy Habits and Sleep Hygiene
S1. Bedtime - No food past 3 hours & only drank water past 2 hours _____
S2. Did a calming routine (e.g., meditation, warm bath, journaling, stating affirmations, expressing gratitude, etc.) _____
S3. Your bed area is device free (your cell phone, tablets, laptops are 5+ feet away and are all turned off) _____
S4. Your room is noise free and dark once lights are off _____
S5. Going to bed early to ensure at least 7 hours of sleep _____
S6. Going to bed around the same time as previous days _____
S7. Finished tracking points in each category today! _____
4 points - good start. 5-6 points - great! 7+ points - excellent! **Total** _____

Notes

_____

_____

_____

_____

_____

_____

_____

_____

Date: _____

Day 4

Give 1 point for each item and add total points for each category
Morning Ritual
Upon waking up, start your day with 1-minute positive mental conditioning exercises
MR1. Write down your affirmation in the present tense 3 times

_____

_____

_____ _____

MR2. Read your affirmation out loud in front a mirror and try to feel excited
MR3. Express gratitude mentally or out loud 3 times. It can be as _____
simple as "Thank you" or "I'm grateful for losing weight"
1 point - good start. 2 points - awesome! 3 points excellent!   **Total** _____

Morning - Healthy Eating Habits
M1. Before you eat or drink, record your weight here _____ lbs   _____

M2. Kickstart your metabolism, regulate your blood sugar, curb cravings - drink 8oz of warm water with
  a). Apple cider vinegar capsules OR
  b). Hand squeezed lemon juice   _____

M3. High-nutrient, low-carb breakfast. Include:

1. Lean protein (eggs, smoked salmon, plant-based protein, etc.)   _____
2. Healthy fats (nuts, nut butter, seeds, avocado)   _____
3. Low-sugar raw fruit (orange, berries, melons, apple)   _____
4. Minimally processed carbs, high in fiber (whole grain/wheat)   _____
Optional: Low-sugar, low fat plant-based milk (almond)   _____
3-4 points - good start. 5-6 points - amazing! 7 points - super!   **Total** _____

Lunch - Healthy Eating Habits
L1. High-nutrient, low-carb lunch salads 5 times each week to fuel your body and curb cravings. Include:

1. Lean proteins (eggs, chicken, beef, fish, tofu, etc.) PLUS _____

2. Leafy greens (arugula, mixed greens) PLUS _____

3. Your favorite vinegarette dressing (apple, strawberry) _____

Optional: Low-sugar fruit (orange, berries, avocado, tomatoes) _____

Optional: Nuts / seeds _____

Optional - You drink low-sodium, low-carb soup (chick broth, miso soup) to help you feel fuller _____

Afternoon - Healthy Snacking Habits
A1. Drink 8 oz of water before snacking to curb cravings _____

A2. High-nutrient, low-calorie snacks – total calorie <300 _____

Optional If you drink non-water beverages, there's no added sugar (For coffee/tea, replace sugar/milk/cream with plant-based milk) _____

4 points - good start. 5-6 points - amazing!

7+ points - you are unstoppable in beating weight gain! **Total** _____

Dinner - Healthy Eating Habits
D1. High-nutrient, low-carb dinner 5 times each week to fuel your body and curb cravings. Include:

1. Lean proteins (eggs, chicken, beef, fish, tofu, etc.) PLUS _____

2. Veggies rich in fiber, minerals, vitamins (green beans, spinach, celery, carrot, bok choy, etc.) _____

3. Minimally processed carbs (brown rice, whole grains) _____

Optional - Fresh fruit as desert _____

Bonus: No carbs or consume 50% less carbs than before _____

Bonus: Only use low-sodium salt / soy sauce for flavor _____

D2. No eating or snacking after 8pm your time _____

3 points - good start. 4-5 points - awesome! 6-7 points - excellent! **Total** _____

Easy Calorie-Burning Habits

CB1. Worked out for 20-30 min and burned 200+ calories
You applied following techniques to prevent your metabolism from plateauing

a). Used more than 1 type of exercise machine _____

b). Varied resistance and/or speed of the machine you used _____

CB2. Instead of going to the gym, you did a 30-min brisk walk or 20-min run or 20-min bike ride _____

CB3. Did a 30-min sport _____

CB4. Drank plenty of water after your exercise _____

CB5. Walked at a moderate speed for 10+ min after lunch _____

CB6. Took the stairs, skipped the elevator _____

CB7. Walked at a moderate speed for 20+ min after dinner _____

Bonus: Did 50 sit-ups and/or 20 push-ups (any style, lazy style) while consuming digital content (e.g., listening to music, pod cast, watching TV) at home _____

Bonus: If you have an adjustable desk at home or work, you stood while worked at your desk for 60+ minutes _____

5 – 6 points - good start. 7 – 8 points – amazing!
9+ points - you are on fire! **Total** _____

Night Time Healthy Habits and Sleep Hygiene

S1. Bedtime - No food past 3 hours & only drank water past 2 hours _____

S2. Did a calming routine (e.g., meditation, warm bath, journaling, stating affirmations, expressing gratitude, etc.) _____

S3. Your bed area is device free (your cell phone, tablets, laptops are 5+ feet away and are all turned off) _____

S4. Your room is noise free and dark once lights are off _____

S5. Going to bed early to ensure at least 7 hours of sleep _____

S6. Going to bed around the same time as previous days _____

S7. Finished tracking points in each category today! _____

4 points - good start. 5-6 points - great! 7+ points - excellent! **Total** _____

Notes

_____

_____

_____

_____

_____

_____

_____

_____

Date: _____

Day 5

➤━━━━━━━━━━━━━━━━━━━━━━━━━━━━➤

Give 1 point for each item and add total points for each category

Morning Ritual

Upon waking up, start your day with 1-minute positive mental conditioning exercises

MR1. Write down your affirmation in the present tense 3 times

_____

_____

_____

MR2. Read your affirmation out loud in front a mirror and try to feel excited

MR3. Express gratitude mentally or out loud 3 times. It can be as simple as "Thank you" or "I'm grateful for losing weight"

1 point - good start. 2 points - awesome! 3 points excellent!   **Total**

Morning - Healthy Eating Habits

M1. Before you eat or drink, record your weight here _____ lbs

M2. Kickstart your metabolism, regulate your blood sugar, curb cravings - drink 8oz of warm water with

   a). Apple cider vinegar capsules OR

   b). Hand squeezed lemon juice

M3. High-nutrient, low-carb breakfast. Include:

1. Lean protein (eggs, smoked salmon, plant-based protein, etc.)
2. Healthy fats (nuts, nut butter, seeds, avocado)
3. Low-sugar raw fruit (orange, berries, melons, apple)
4. Minimally processed carbs, high in fiber (whole grain/wheat)

Optional: Low-sugar, low fat plant-based milk (almond)

3-4 points - good start. 5-6 points - amazing! 7 points - super!   **Total**

Lunch - Healthy Eating Habits

L1. High-nutrient, low-carb lunch salads 5 times each week to fuel your body and curb cravings. Include:

1. Lean proteins (eggs, chicken, beef, fish, tofu, etc.) PLUS _____

2. Leafy greens (arugula, mixed greens) PLUS _____

3. Your favorite vinegarette dressing (apple, strawberry) _____

Optional: Low-sugar fruit (orange, berries, avocado, tomatoes) _____

Optional: Nuts / seeds _____

Optional - You drink low-sodium, low-carb soup (chick broth, miso soup) to help you feel fuller _____

Afternoon - Healthy Snacking Habits

A1. Drink 8 oz of water before snacking to curb cravings _____

A2. High-nutrient, low-calorie snacks – total calorie <300 _____

Optional If you drink non-water beverages, there's no added sugar (For coffee/tea, replace sugar/milk/cream with plant-based milk) _____

4 points - good start. 5-6 points - amazing!

7+ points - you are unstoppable in beating weight gain! **Total** _____

Dinner - Healthy Eating Habits

D1. High-nutrient, low-carb dinner 5 times each week to fuel your body and curb cravings. Include:

1. Lean proteins (eggs, chicken, beef, fish, tofu, etc.) PLUS _____

2. Veggies rich in fiber, minerals, vitamins (green beans, spinach, celery, carrot, bok choy, etc.) _____

3. Minimally processed carbs (brown rice, whole grains) _____

Optional - Fresh fruit as desert _____

Bonus: No carbs or consume 50% less carbs than before _____

Bonus: Only use low-sodium salt / soy sauce for flavor _____

D2. No eating or snacking after 8pm your time _____

3 points - good start. 4-5 points - awesome! 6-7 points - excellent! **Total** _____

Easy Calorie-Burning Habits
CB1. Worked out for 20-30 min and burned 200+ calories
You applied following techniques to prevent your metabolism from plateauing
a). Used more than 1 type of exercise machine _____
b). Varied resistance and/or speed of the machine you used _____
CB2. Instead of going to the gym, you did a 30-min brisk walk or 20-min run or 20-min bike ride _____
CB3. Did a 30-min sport _____
CB4. Drank plenty of water after your exercise _____
CB5. Walked at a moderate speed for 10+ min after lunch _____
CB6. Took the stairs, skipped the elevator _____
CB7. Walked at a moderate speed for 20+ min after dinner _____
Bonus: Did 50 sit-ups and/or 20 push-ups (any style, lazy style) while consuming digital content (e.g., listening to music, pod cast, watching TV) at home _____
Bonus: If you have an adjustable desk at home or work, you stood while worked at your desk for 60+ minutes _____
5 – 6 points - good start. 7 – 8 points – amazing!
9+ points - you are on fire!   **Total** _____

Night Time Healthy Habits and Sleep Hygiene
S1. Bedtime - No food past 3 hours & only drank water past 2 hours _____
S2. Did a calming routine (e.g., meditation, warm bath, journaling, stating affirmations, expressing gratitude, etc.) _____
S3. Your bed area is device free (your cell phone, tablets, laptops are 5+ feet away and are all turned off) _____
S4. Your room is noise free and dark once lights are off _____
S5. Going to bed early to ensure at least 7 hours of sleep _____
S6. Going to bed around the same time as previous days _____
S7. Finished tracking points in each category today! _____
4 points - good start. 5-6 points - great! 7+ points - excellent!   **Total** _____

Notes

Date: _____

Day 6

Give 1 point for each item and add total points for each category

Morning Ritual

Upon waking up, start your day with 1-minute positive mental conditioning exercises

MR1. Write down your affirmation in the present tense 3 times

_____

_____

_____ _____

MR2. Read your affirmation out loud in front a mirror and try to feel excited   _____

MR3. Express gratitude mentally or out loud 3 times. It can be as simple as "Thank you" or "I'm grateful for losing weight"   _____

1 point - good start. 2 points - awesome! 3 points excellent!   **Total** ▬▬▬

Morning - Healthy Eating Habits

M1. Before you eat or drink, record your weight here _____ lbs   _____

M2. Kickstart your metabolism, regulate your blood sugar, curb cravings - drink 8oz of warm water with

   a). Apple cider vinegar capsules OR

   b). Hand squeezed lemon juice   _____

M3. High-nutrient, low-carb breakfast. Include:

1. Lean protein (eggs, smoked salmon, plant-based protein, etc.)   _____
2. Healthy fats (nuts, nut butter, seeds, avocado)   _____
3. Low-sugar raw fruit (orange, berries, melons, apple)   _____
4. Minimally processed carbs, high in fiber (whole grain/wheat)   _____

Optional: Low-sugar, low fat plant-based milk (almond)   _____

3-4 points - good start. 5-6 points - amazing! 7 points - super!   **Total** ▬▬▬

Lunch - Healthy Eating Habits

L1. High-nutrient, low-carb lunch salads 5 times each week to fuel your body and curb cravings. Include:

1. Lean proteins (eggs, chicken, beef, fish, tofu, etc.) PLUS _____

2. Leafy greens (arugula, mixed greens) PLUS _____

3. Your favorite vinegarette dressing (apple, strawberry) _____

Optional: Low-sugar fruit (orange, berries, avocado, tomatoes) _____

Optional: Nuts / seeds _____

Optional - You drink low-sodium, low-carb soup (chick broth, miso soup) to help you feel fuller _____

Afternoon - Healthy Snacking Habits

A1. Drink 8 oz of water before snacking to curb cravings _____

A2. High-nutrient, low-calorie snacks – total calorie <300 _____

Optional If you drink non-water beverages, there's no added sugar (For coffee/tea, replace sugar/milk/cream with plant-based milk) _____

4 points - good start. 5-6 points - amazing!

7+ points - you are unstoppable in beating weight gain! **Total** _____

Dinner - Healthy Eating Habits

D1. High-nutrient, low-carb dinner 5 times each week to fuel your body and curb cravings. Include:

1. Lean proteins (eggs, chicken, beef, fish, tofu, etc.) PLUS _____

2. Veggies rich in fiber, minerals, vitamins (green beans, spinach, celery, carrot, bok choy, etc.) _____

3. Minimally processed carbs (brown rice, whole grains) _____

Optional - Fresh fruit as desert _____

Bonus: No carbs or consume 50% less carbs than before _____

Bonus: Only use low-sodium salt / soy sauce for flavor _____

D2. No eating or snacking after 8pm your time _____

3 points - good start. 4-5 points - awesome! 6-7 points - excellent! **Total** _____

Easy Calorie-Burning Habits

CB1. Worked out for 20-30 min and burned 200+ calories
You applied following techniques to prevent your metabolism from plateauing
a). Used more than 1 type of exercise machine _____
b). Varied resistance and/or speed of the machine you used _____
CB2. Instead of going to the gym, you did a 30-min brisk walk or 20-min run or 20-min bike ride _____
CB3. Did a 30-min sport _____
CB4. Drank plenty of water after your exercise _____
CB5. Walked at a moderate speed for 10+ min after lunch _____
CB6. Took the stairs, skipped the elevator _____
CB7. Walked at a moderate speed for 20+ min after dinner _____
Bonus: Did 50 sit-ups and/or 20 push-ups (any style, lazy style) while consuming digital content (e.g., listening to music, pod cast, watching TV) at home
Bonus: If you have an adjustable desk at home or work, you stood while worked at your desk for 60+ minutes _____
5 – 6 points - good start. 7 – 8 points – amazing!
9+ points - you are on fire! **Total** _____

Night Time Healthy Habits and Sleep Hygiene

S1. Bedtime - No food past 3 hours & only drank water past 2 hours _____
S2. Did a calming routine (e.g., meditation, warm bath, journaling, stating affirmations, expressing gratitude, etc.) _____
S3. Your bed area is device free (your cell phone, tablets, laptops are 5+ feet away and are all turned off) _____
S4. Your room is noise free and dark once lights are off _____
S5. Going to bed early to ensure at least 7 hours of sleep _____
S6. Going to bed around the same time as previous days _____
S7. Finished tracking points in each category today! _____
4 points - good start. 5-6 points - great! 7+ points - excellent! **Total** _____

Notes

Date: _____

Day 7

Give 1 point for each item and add total points for each category

Morning Ritual

Upon waking up, start your day with 1-minute positive mental conditioning exercises

MR1. Write down your affirmation in the present tense 3 times

_____

_____

_____   _____

MR2. Read your affirmation out loud in front a mirror and try to feel excited

MR3. Express gratitude mentally or out loud 3 times. It can be as simple as "Thank you" or "I'm grateful for losing weight"   _____

1 point - good start. 2 points - awesome! 3 points excellent!   **Total**   _____

Morning - Healthy Eating Habits

M1. Before you eat or drink, record your weight here _____ lbs   _____

M2. Kickstart your metabolism, regulate your blood sugar, curb cravings - drink 8oz of warm water with
   a). Apple cider vinegar capsules OR
   b). Hand squeezed lemon juice   _____

M3. High-nutrient, low-carb breakfast. Include:

1. Lean protein (eggs, smoked salmon, plant-based protein, etc.)   _____
2. Healthy fats (nuts, nut butter, seeds, avocado)   _____
3. Low-sugar raw fruit (orange, berries, melons, apple)   _____
4. Minimally processed carbs, high in fiber (whole grain/wheat)   _____
Optional: Low-sugar, low fat plant-based milk (almond)   _____
3-4 points - good start. 5-6 points - amazing! 7 points - super!   **Total**   _____

Lunch - Healthy Eating Habits

L1. High-nutrient, low-carb lunch salads 5 times each week to fuel your body and curb cravings. Include:

1. Lean proteins (eggs, chicken, beef, fish, tofu, etc.) PLUS

2. Leafy greens (arugula, mixed greens) PLUS

3. Your favorite vinegarette dressing (apple, strawberry)

Optional: Low-sugar fruit (orange, berries, avocado, tomatoes)

Optional: Nuts / seeds

Optional - You drink low-sodium, low-carb soup (chick broth, miso soup) to help you feel fuller

Afternoon - Healthy Snacking Habits

A1. Drink 8 oz of water before snacking to curb cravings

A2. High-nutrient, low-calorie snacks – total calorie <300

Optional If you drink non-water beverages, there's no added sugar (For coffee/tea, replace sugar/milk/cream with plant-based milk)

4 points - good start. 5-6 points - amazing!

7+ points - you are unstoppable in beating weight gain!   **Total**

Dinner - Healthy Eating Habits

D1. High-nutrient, low-carb dinner 5 times each week to fuel your body and curb cravings. Include:

1. Lean proteins (eggs, chicken, beef, fish, tofu, etc.) PLUS

2. Veggies rich in fiber, minerals, vitamins (green beans, spinach, celery, carrot, bok choy, etc.)

3. Minimally processed carbs (brown rice, whole grains)

Optional - Fresh fruit as desert

Bonus: No carbs or consume 50% less carbs than before

Bonus: Only use low-sodium salt / soy sauce for flavor

D2. No eating or snacking after 8pm your time

3 points - good start. 4-5 points - awesome! 6-7 points - excellent!   **Total**

Easy Calorie-Burning Habits

CB1. Worked out for 20-30 min and burned 200+ calories

You applied following techniques to prevent your metabolism from plateauing

a). Used more than 1 type of exercise machine

b). Varied resistance and/or speed of the machine you used _____

CB2. Instead of going to the gym, you did a 30-min brisk walk or 20-min run or 20-min bike ride _____

CB3. Did a 30-min sport _____

CB4. Drank plenty of water after your exercise _____

CB5. Walked at a moderate speed for 10+ min after lunch _____

CB6. Took the stairs, skipped the elevator _____

CB7. Walked at a moderate speed for 20+ min after dinner _____

Bonus: Did 50 sit-ups and/or 20 push-ups (any style, lazy style) while consuming digital content (e.g., listening to music, pod cast, watching TV) at home _____

Bonus: If you have an adjustable desk at home or work, you stood while worked at your desk for 60+ minutes _____

5 – 6 points - good start. 7 – 8 points – amazing!

9+ points - you are on fire!   **Total** _____

Night Time Healthy Habits and Sleep Hygiene

S1. Bedtime - No food past 3 hours & only drank water past 2 hours _____

S2. Did a calming routine (e.g., meditation, warm bath, journaling, stating affirmations, expressing gratitude, etc.) _____

S3. Your bed area is device free (your cell phone, tablets, laptops are 5+ feet away and are all turned off) _____

S4. Your room is noise free and dark once lights are off _____

S5. Going to bed early to ensure at least 7 hours of sleep _____

S6. Going to bed around the same time as previous days _____

S7. Finished tracking points in each category today! _____

4 points - good start. 5-6 points - great! 7+ points - excellent!   **Total** _____

Notes

Date: _____

End of Week 2 Reflection

Day 1 weight _____   Day 7 weight _____

Which habit categories you ...	...consistently scored well?	...consistently scored lower (good start)?	...plan to improve the most next week?
Morning Ritual			
Morning Healthy Eating Habits			
Lunch Healthy Eating + Afternoon Healthy Snacking Habits			
Dinner Healthy Eating Habits			
Calorie-Burning Habits			
Night Time Healthy Habits and Sleep Hygiene			

Pat yourself on the back even if your weight roughly stayed the same this week. The fact that you have completed this entire week's habit tracking is a win! Celebrate every win, small or big. Just don't binge-eat your guilty pleasures. Take everything in moderation and you will see and feel the rewards of living a healthy lifestyle.

If your weight increases, which could very well be water retention caused by menstruation, high-sodium foods, or high-carb foods, continue the daily habits next week. As long as you try to improve the categories you scored low this week, you will see tangible weight loss soon.

State these gratitude statements out loud 3 times and try to feel your weight loss outcomes and get excited:

- I am so grateful for feeling lighter, leaner and more energetic!
- I am so grateful for completing daily habit tracking.
- I am so grateful for putting high-nutrient foods in my body and keeping myself active.

Week 3

Date: _____

Day 1

Give 1 point for each item and add total points for each category

Morning Ritual

Upon waking up, start your day with 1-minute positive mental conditioning exercises

MR1. Write down your affirmation in the present tense 3 times

_____

_____

_____ _____

MR2. Read your affirmation out loud in front a mirror and try to feel excited _____

MR3. Express gratitude mentally or out loud 3 times. It can be as simple as "Thank you" or "I'm grateful for losing weight" _____

1 point - good start. 2 points - awesome! 3 points excellent!   **Total** _____

Morning - Healthy Eating Habits

M1. Before you eat or drink, record your weight here _____ lbs _____

M2. Kickstart your metabolism, regulate your blood sugar, curb cravings - drink 8oz of warm water with
  a). Apple cider vinegar capsules OR
  b). Hand squeezed lemon juice _____

M3. High-nutrient, low-carb breakfast. Include:

1. Lean protein (eggs, smoked salmon, plant-based protein, etc.) _____
2. Healthy fats (nuts, nut butter, seeds, avocado) _____
3. Low-sugar raw fruit (orange, berries, melons, apple) _____
4. Minimally processed carbs, high in fiber (whole grain/wheat) _____
Optional: Low-sugar, low fat plant-based milk (almond) _____

3-4 points - good start. 5-6 points - amazing! 7 points - super!   **Total** _____

Lunch - Healthy Eating Habits

L1. High-nutrient, low-carb lunch salads 5 times each week to fuel your body and curb cravings. Include:

1. Lean proteins (eggs, chicken, beef, fish, tofu, etc.) PLUS _____

2. Leafy greens (arugula, mixed greens) PLUS _____

3. Your favorite vinegarette dressing (apple, strawberry) _____

Optional: Low-sugar fruit (orange, berries, avocado, tomatoes) _____

Optional: Nuts / seeds _____

Optional - You drink low-sodium, low-carb soup (chick broth, miso soup) to help you feel fuller _____

Afternoon - Healthy Snacking Habits

A1. Drink 8 oz of water before snacking to curb cravings _____

A2. High-nutrient, low-calorie snacks – total calorie <300 _____

Optional If you drink non-water beverages, there's no added sugar (For coffee/tea, replace sugar/milk/cream with plant-based milk) _____

4 points - good start. 5-6 points - amazing!

7+ points - you are unstoppable in beating weight gain! **Total** _____

Dinner - Healthy Eating Habits

D1. High-nutrient, low-carb dinner 5 times each week to fuel your body and curb cravings. Include:

1. Lean proteins (eggs, chicken, beef, fish, tofu, etc.) PLUS _____

2. Veggies rich in fiber, minerals, vitamins (green beans, spinach, celery, carrot, bok choy, etc.) _____

3. Minimally processed carbs (brown rice, whole grains) _____

Optional - Fresh fruit as desert _____

Bonus: No carbs or consume 50% less carbs than before _____

Bonus: Only use low-sodium salt / soy sauce for flavor _____

D2. No eating or snacking after 8pm your time _____

3 points - good start. 4-5 points - awesome! 6-7 points - excellent! **Total** _____

Easy Calorie-Burning Habits
CB1. Worked out for 20-30 min and burned 200+ calories
You applied following techniques to prevent your metabolism from plateauing
a). Used more than 1 type of exercise machine
b). Varied resistance and/or speed of the machine you used _____
CB2. Instead of going to the gym, you did a 30-min brisk walk or 20-min run or 20-min bike ride
CB3. Did a 30-min sport _____
CB4. Drank plenty of water after your exercise _____
CB5. Walked at a moderate speed for 10+ min after lunch _____
CB6. Took the stairs, skipped the elevator _____
CB7. Walked at a moderate speed for 20+ min after dinner _____
Bonus: Did 50 sit-ups and/or 20 push-ups (any style, lazy style) while consuming digital content (e.g., listening to music, pod cast, watching TV) at home _____
Bonus: If you have an adjustable desk at home or work, you stood while worked at your desk for 60+ minutes _____
5 – 6 points - good start. 7 – 8 points – amazing!
9+ points - you are on fire! **Total** _____

Night Time Healthy Habits and Sleep Hygiene
S1. Bedtime - No food past 3 hours & only drank water past 2 hours _____
S2. Did a calming routine (e.g., meditation, warm bath, journaling, stating affirmations, expressing gratitude, etc.) _____
S3. Your bed area is device free (your cell phone, tablets, laptops are 5+ feet away and are all turned off) _____
S4. Your room is noise free and dark once lights are off _____
S5. Going to bed early to ensure at least 7 hours of sleep _____
S6. Going to bed around the same time as previous days _____
S7. Finished tracking points in each category today! _____
4 points - good start. 5-6 points - great! 7+ points - excellent! **Total** _____

Notes

Date: _____

Day 2

Give 1 point for each item and add total points for each category

Morning Ritual

Upon waking up, start your day with 1-minute positive mental conditioning exercises

MR1. Write down your affirmation in the present tense 3 times

_____

_____

_____   _____

MR2. Read your affirmation out loud in front a mirror and try to feel excited   _____

MR3. Express gratitude mentally or out loud 3 times. It can be as simple as "Thank you" or "I'm grateful for losing weight"   _____

1 point - good start. 2 points - awesome! 3 points excellent!   **Total**   _____

Morning - Healthy Eating Habits

M1. Before you eat or drink, record your weight here _____ lbs   _____

M2. Kickstart your metabolism, regulate your blood sugar, curb cravings - drink 8oz of warm water with
   a). Apple cider vinegar capsules OR
   b). Hand squeezed lemon juice   _____

M3. High-nutrient, low-carb breakfast. Include:

1. Lean protein (eggs, smoked salmon, plant-based protein, etc.)   _____
2. Healthy fats (nuts, nut butter, seeds, avocado)   _____
3. Low-sugar raw fruit (orange, berries, melons, apple)   _____
4. Minimally processed carbs, high in fiber (whole grain/wheat)   _____
Optional: Low-sugar, low fat plant-based milk (almond)   _____
3-4 points - good start. 5-6 points - amazing! 7 points - super!   **Total**   _____

Lunch - Healthy Eating Habits

L1. High-nutrient, low-carb lunch salads 5 times each week to fuel your body and curb cravings. Include:

1. Lean proteins (eggs, chicken, beef, fish, tofu, etc.) PLUS _____

2. Leafy greens (arugula, mixed greens) PLUS _____

3. Your favorite vinegarette dressing (apple, strawberry) _____

Optional: Low-sugar fruit (orange, berries, avocado, tomatoes) _____

Optional: Nuts / seeds _____

Optional - You drink low-sodium, low-carb soup (chick broth, miso soup) to help you feel fuller _____

Afternoon - Healthy Snacking Habits

A1. Drink 8 oz of water before snacking to curb cravings _____

A2. High-nutrient, low-calorie snacks – total calorie <300 _____

Optional If you drink non-water beverages, there's no added sugar (For coffee/tea, replace sugar/milk/cream with plant-based milk) _____

4 points - good start. 5-6 points - amazing!

7+ points - you are unstoppable in beating weight gain!   **Total** _____

Dinner - Healthy Eating Habits

D1. High-nutrient, low-carb dinner 5 times each week to fuel your body and curb cravings. Include:

1. Lean proteins (eggs, chicken, beef, fish, tofu, etc.) PLUS _____

2. Veggies rich in fiber, minerals, vitamins (green beans, spinach, celery, carrot, bok choy, etc.) _____

3. Minimally processed carbs (brown rice, whole grains) _____

Optional - Fresh fruit as desert _____

Bonus: No carbs or consume 50% less carbs than before _____

Bonus: Only use low-sodium salt / soy sauce for flavor _____

D2. No eating or snacking after 8pm your time _____

3 points - good start. 4-5 points - awesome! 6-7 points - excellent!   **Total** _____

Easy Calorie-Burning Habits
CB1. Worked out for 20-30 min and burned 200+ calories
You applied following techniques to prevent your metabolism from plateauing
a). Used more than 1 type of exercise machine   _____
b). Varied resistance and/or speed of the machine you used   _____
CB2. Instead of going to the gym, you did a 30-min brisk walk or 20-min run or 20-min bike ride
CB3. Did a 30-min sport   _____
CB4. Drank plenty of water after your exercise   _____
CB5. Walked at a moderate speed for 10+ min after lunch   _____
CB6. Took the stairs, skipped the elevator   _____
CB7. Walked at a moderate speed for 20+ min after dinner   _____
Bonus: Did 50 sit-ups and/or 20 push-ups (any style, lazy style) while consuming digital content (e.g., listening to music, pod cast, watching TV) at home   _____
Bonus: If you have an adjustable desk at home or work, you stood while worked at your desk for 60+ minutes   _____
5 – 6 points - good start. 7 – 8 points – amazing!
9+ points - you are on fire!   **Total** _____

Night Time Healthy Habits and Sleep Hygiene
S1. Bedtime - No food past 3 hours & only drank water past 2 hours   _____
S2. Did a calming routine (e.g., meditation, warm bath, journaling, stating affirmations, expressing gratitude, etc.)   _____
S3. Your bed area is device free (your cell phone, tablets, laptops are 5+ feet away and are all turned off)   _____
S4. Your room is noise free and dark once lights are off   _____
S5. Going to bed early to ensure at least 7 hours of sleep   _____
S6. Going to bed around the same time as previous days   _____
S7. Finished tracking points in each category today!   _____
4 points - good start. 5-6 points - great! 7+ points - excellent! **Total** _____

Notes

Date: _____

Day 3

Give 1 point for each item and add total points for each category

Morning Ritual

Upon waking up, start your day with 1-minute positive mental conditioning exercises

MR1. Write down your affirmation in the present tense 3 times

_____

_____

_____   _____

MR2. Read your affirmation out loud in front a mirror and try to feel excited   _____

MR3. Express gratitude mentally or out loud 3 times. It can be as simple as "Thank you" or "I'm grateful for losing weight"   _____

1 point - good start. 2 points - awesome! 3 points excellent!   **Total** _____

Morning - Healthy Eating Habits

M1. Before you eat or drink, record your weight here _____ lbs   _____

M2. Kickstart your metabolism, regulate your blood sugar, curb cravings - drink 8oz of warm water with

    a). Apple cider vinegar capsules OR

    b). Hand squeezed lemon juice   _____

M3. High-nutrient, low-carb breakfast. Include:

1. Lean protein (eggs, smoked salmon, plant-based protein, etc.)   _____
2. Healthy fats (nuts, nut butter, seeds, avocado)   _____
3. Low-sugar raw fruit (orange, berries, melons, apple)   _____
4. Minimally processed carbs, high in fiber (whole grain/wheat)   _____
Optional: Low-sugar, low fat plant-based milk (almond)   _____

3-4 points - good start. 5-6 points - amazing! 7 points - super!   **Total** _____

Lunch - Healthy Eating Habits

L1. High-nutrient, low-carb lunch salads 5 times each week to fuel your body and curb cravings. Include:

1. Lean proteins (eggs, chicken, beef, fish, tofu, etc.) PLUS   _____

2. Leafy greens (arugula, mixed greens) PLUS   _____

3. Your favorite vinegarette dressing (apple, strawberry)   _____

Optional: Low-sugar fruit (orange, berries, avocado, tomatoes)   _____

Optional: Nuts / seeds   _____

Optional - You drink low-sodium, low-carb soup (chick broth, miso soup) to help you feel fuller   _____

Afternoon - Healthy Snacking Habits

A1. Drink 8 oz of water before snacking to curb cravings   _____

A2. High-nutrient, low-calorie snacks – total calorie <300   _____

Optional If you drink non-water beverages, there's no added sugar (For coffee/tea, replace sugar/milk/cream with plant-based milk)   _____

4 points - good start. 5-6 points - amazing!

7+ points - you are unstoppable in beating weight gain!   **Total** _____

Dinner - Healthy Eating Habits

D1. High-nutrient, low-carb dinner 5 times each week to fuel your body and curb cravings. Include:

1. Lean proteins (eggs, chicken, beef, fish, tofu, etc.) PLUS   _____

2. Veggies rich in fiber, minerals, vitamins (green beans, spinach, celery, carrot, bok choy, etc.)   _____

3. Minimally processed carbs (brown rice, whole grains)   _____

Optional - Fresh fruit as desert   _____

Bonus: No carbs or consume 50% less carbs than before   _____

Bonus: Only use low-sodium salt / soy sauce for flavor   _____

D2. No eating or snacking after 8pm your time

3 points - good start. 4-5 points - awesome! 6-7 points - excellent!   **Total** _____

Easy Calorie-Burning Habits

CB1. Worked out for 20-30 min and burned 200+ calories

You applied following techniques to prevent your metabolism from plateauing

a). Used more than 1 type of exercise machine _____

b). Varied resistance and/or speed of the machine you used _____

CB2. Instead of going to the gym, you did a 30-min brisk walk or 20-min run or 20-min bike ride _____

CB3. Did a 30-min sport _____

CB4. Drank plenty of water after your exercise _____

CB5. Walked at a moderate speed for 10+ min after lunch _____

CB6. Took the stairs, skipped the elevator _____

CB7. Walked at a moderate speed for 20+ min after dinner _____

Bonus: Did 50 sit-ups and/or 20 push-ups (any style, lazy style) while consuming digital content (e.g., listening to music, pod cast, watching TV) at home _____

Bonus: If you have an adjustable desk at home or work, you stood while worked at your desk for 60+ minutes _____

5 – 6 points - good start. 7 – 8 points – amazing!

9+ points - you are on fire!   **Total** _____

Night Time Healthy Habits and Sleep Hygiene

S1. Bedtime - No food past 3 hours & only drank water past 2 hours _____

S2. Did a calming routine (e.g., meditation, warm bath, journaling, stating affirmations, expressing gratitude, etc.) _____

S3. Your bed area is device free (your cell phone, tablets, laptops are 5+ feet away and are all turned off) _____

S4. Your room is noise free and dark once lights are off _____

S5. Going to bed early to ensure at least 7 hours of sleep _____

S6. Going to bed around the same time as previous days _____

S7. Finished tracking points in each category today! _____

4 points - good start. 5-6 points - great! 7+ points - excellent!   **Total** _____

Notes

Date: _____

Day 4

Give 1 point for each item and add total points for each category

Morning Ritual

Upon waking up, start your day with 1-minute positive mental conditioning exercises

MR1. Write down your affirmation in the present tense 3 times

_____

_____

_____   _____

MR2. Read your affirmation out loud in front a mirror and try to feel excited   _____

MR3. Express gratitude mentally or out loud 3 times. It can be as simple as "Thank you" or "I'm grateful for losing weight"   _____

1 point - good start. 2 points - awesome! 3 points excellent!   **Total**   _____

Morning - Healthy Eating Habits

M1. Before you eat or drink, record your weight here _____ lbs   _____

M2. Kickstart your metabolism, regulate your blood sugar, curb cravings - drink 8oz of warm water with

   a). Apple cider vinegar capsules OR

   b). Hand squeezed lemon juice   _____

M3. High-nutrient, low-carb breakfast. Include:

1. Lean protein (eggs, smoked salmon, plant-based protein, etc.)   _____
2. Healthy fats (nuts, nut butter, seeds, avocado)   _____
3. Low-sugar raw fruit (orange, berries, melons, apple)   _____
4. Minimally processed carbs, high in fiber (whole grain/wheat)   _____

Optional: Low-sugar, low fat plant-based milk (almond)   _____

3-4 points - good start. 5-6 points - amazing! 7 points - super!   **Total**   _____

Lunch - Healthy Eating Habits

L1. High-nutrient, low-carb lunch salads 5 times each week to fuel your body and curb cravings. Include:

1. Lean proteins (eggs, chicken, beef, fish, tofu, etc.) PLUS _____

2. Leafy greens (arugula, mixed greens) PLUS _____

3. Your favorite vinegarette dressing (apple, strawberry) _____

Optional: Low-sugar fruit (orange, berries, avocado, tomatoes) _____

Optional: Nuts / seeds _____

Optional - You drink low-sodium, low-carb soup (chick broth, miso soup) to help you feel fuller _____

Afternoon - Healthy Snacking Habits

A1. Drink 8 oz of water before snacking to curb cravings _____

A2. High-nutrient, low-calorie snacks – total calorie <300 _____

Optional If you drink non-water beverages, there's no added sugar (For coffee/tea, replace sugar/milk/cream with plant-based milk) _____

4 points - good start. 5-6 points - amazing!

7+ points - you are unstoppable in beating weight gain!   **Total** _____

Dinner - Healthy Eating Habits

D1. High-nutrient, low-carb dinner 5 times each week to fuel your body and curb cravings. Include:

1. Lean proteins (eggs, chicken, beef, fish, tofu, etc.) PLUS _____

2. Veggies rich in fiber, minerals, vitamins (green beans, spinach, celery, carrot, bok choy, etc.) _____

3. Minimally processed carbs (brown rice, whole grains) _____

Optional - Fresh fruit as desert _____

Bonus: No carbs or consume 50% less carbs than before _____

Bonus: Only use low-sodium salt / soy sauce for flavor _____

D2. No eating or snacking after 8pm your time _____

3 points - good start. 4-5 points - awesome! 6-7 points - excellent!   **Total** _____

Easy Calorie-Burning Habits

CB1. Worked out for 20-30 min and burned 200+ calories
You applied following techniques to prevent your metabolism from plateauing
a). Used more than 1 type of exercise machine _____
b). Varied resistance and/or speed of the machine you used _____
CB2. Instead of going to the gym, you did a 30-min brisk walk or 20-min run or 20-min bike ride _____
CB3. Did a 30-min sport _____
CB4. Drank plenty of water after your exercise _____
CB5. Walked at a moderate speed for 10+ min after lunch _____
CB6. Took the stairs, skipped the elevator _____
CB7. Walked at a moderate speed for 20+ min after dinner _____
Bonus: Did 50 sit-ups and/or 20 push-ups (any style, lazy style) while consuming digital content (e.g., listening to music, pod cast, watching TV) at home _____
Bonus: If you have an adjustable desk at home or work, you stood while worked at your desk for 60+ minutes _____
5 – 6 points - good start. 7 – 8 points – amazing!
9+ points - you are on fire! **Total** _____

Night Time Healthy Habits and Sleep Hygiene

S1. Bedtime - No food past 3 hours & only drank water past 2 hours _____
S2. Did a calming routine (e.g., meditation, warm bath, journaling, stating affirmations, expressing gratitude, etc.) _____
S3. Your bed area is device free (your cell phone, tablets, laptops are 5+ feet away and are all turned off) _____
S4. Your room is noise free and dark once lights are off _____
S5. Going to bed early to ensure at least 7 hours of sleep _____
S6. Going to bed around the same time as previous days _____
S7. Finished tracking points in each category today! _____
4 points - good start. 5-6 points - great! 7+ points - excellent! **Total** _____

Notes

Date: _____

Day 5

Give 1 point for each item and add total points for each category
Morning Ritual
Upon waking up, start your day with 1-minute positive mental conditioning exercises
MR1. Write down your affirmation in the present tense 3 times

_____

_____

_____   _____

MR2. Read your affirmation out loud in front a mirror and try to feel excited
MR3. Express gratitude mentally or out loud 3 times. It can be as simple as "Thank you" or "I'm grateful for losing weight"   _____
1 point - good start. 2 points - awesome! 3 points excellent!   **Total** _____

Morning - Healthy Eating Habits
M1. Before you eat or drink, record your weight here _____ lbs   _____

M2. Kickstart your metabolism, regulate your blood sugar, curb cravings - drink 8oz of warm water with
  a). Apple cider vinegar capsules OR
  b). Hand squeezed lemon juice   _____

M3. High-nutrient, low-carb breakfast. Include:

1. Lean protein (eggs, smoked salmon, plant-based protein, etc.)   _____
2. Healthy fats (nuts, nut butter, seeds, avocado)   _____
3. Low-sugar raw fruit (orange, berries, melons, apple)   _____
4. Minimally processed carbs, high in fiber (whole grain/wheat)   _____
Optional: Low-sugar, low fat plant-based milk (almond)   _____
3-4 points - good start. 5-6 points - amazing! 7 points - super! **Total** _____

Lunch - Healthy Eating Habits

L1. High-nutrient, low-carb lunch salads 5 times each week to fuel your body and curb cravings. Include:

1. Lean proteins (eggs, chicken, beef, fish, tofu, etc.) PLUS   _____

2. Leafy greens (arugula, mixed greens) PLUS   _____

3. Your favorite vinegarette dressing (apple, strawberry)   _____

Optional: Low-sugar fruit (orange, berries, avocado, tomatoes)   _____

Optional: Nuts / seeds   _____

Optional - You drink low-sodium, low-carb soup (chick broth, miso soup) to help you feel fuller   _____

Afternoon - Healthy Snacking Habits

A1. Drink 8 oz of water before snacking to curb cravings   _____

A2. High-nutrient, low-calorie snacks – total calorie <300   _____

Optional If you drink non-water beverages, there's no added sugar (For coffee/tea, replace sugar/milk/cream with plant-based milk)   _____

4 points - good start. 5-6 points - amazing!
7+ points - you are unstoppable in beating weight gain!   **Total** _____

Dinner - Healthy Eating Habits

D1. High-nutrient, low-carb dinner 5 times each week to fuel your body and curb cravings. Include:

1. Lean proteins (eggs, chicken, beef, fish, tofu, etc.) PLUS   _____

2. Veggies rich in fiber, minerals, vitamins (green beans, spinach, celery, carrot, bok choy, etc.)   _____

3. Minimally processed carbs (brown rice, whole grains)   _____

Optional - Fresh fruit as desert   _____

Bonus: No carbs or consume 50% less carbs than before   _____

Bonus: Only use low-sodium salt / soy sauce for flavor   _____

D2. No eating or snacking after 8pm your time   _____

3 points - good start. 4-5 points - awesome! 6-7 points - excellent!   **Total** _____

Easy Calorie-Burning Habits

CB1. Worked out for 20-30 min and burned 200+ calories

You applied following techniques to prevent your metabolism from plateauing

a). Used more than 1 type of exercise machine _____

b). Varied resistance and/or speed of the machine you used _____

CB2. Instead of going to the gym, you did a 30-min brisk walk or 20-min run or 20-min bike ride

CB3. Did a 30-min sport _____

CB4. Drank plenty of water after your exercise _____

CB5. Walked at a moderate speed for 10+ min after lunch _____

CB6. Took the stairs, skipped the elevator _____

CB7. Walked at a moderate speed for 20+ min after dinner _____

Bonus: Did 50 sit-ups and/or 20 push-ups (any style, lazy style) while consuming digital content (e.g., listening to music, pod cast, watching TV) at home _____

Bonus: If you have an adjustable desk at home or work, you stood while worked at your desk for 60+ minutes _____

5 – 6 points - good start. 7 – 8 points – amazing!

9+ points - you are on fire! **Total** _____

Night Time Healthy Habits and Sleep Hygiene

S1. Bedtime - No food past 3 hours & only drank water past 2 hours _____

S2. Did a calming routine (e.g., meditation, warm bath, journaling, stating affirmations, expressing gratitude, etc.) _____

S3. Your bed area is device free (your cell phone, tablets, laptops are 5+ feet away and are all turned off)

S4. Your room is noise free and dark once lights are off _____

S5. Going to bed early to ensure at least 7 hours of sleep _____

S6. Going to bed around the same time as previous days _____

S7. Finished tracking points in each category today! _____

4 points - good start. 5-6 points - great! 7+ points - excellent! **Total** _____

Notes

Date: _____

Day 6

Give 1 point for each item and add total points for each category

Morning Ritual

Upon waking up, start your day with 1-minute positive mental conditioning exercises

MR1. Write down your affirmation in the present tense 3 times

_____

_____

_____

MR2. Read your affirmation out loud in front a mirror and try to feel excited

MR3. Express gratitude mentally or out loud 3 times. It can be as simple as "Thank you" or "I'm grateful for losing weight"

1 point - good start. 2 points - awesome! 3 points excellent! **Total**

Morning - Healthy Eating Habits

M1. Before you eat or drink, record your weight here _____ lbs

M2. Kickstart your metabolism, regulate your blood sugar, curb cravings - drink 8oz of warm water with

   a). Apple cider vinegar capsules OR

   b). Hand squeezed lemon juice

M3. High-nutrient, low-carb breakfast. Include:

1. Lean protein (eggs, smoked salmon, plant-based protein, etc.)
2. Healthy fats (nuts, nut butter, seeds, avocado)
3. Low-sugar raw fruit (orange, berries, melons, apple)
4. Minimally processed carbs, high in fiber (whole grain/wheat)

Optional: Low-sugar, low fat plant-based milk (almond)

3-4 points - good start. 5-6 points - amazing! 7 points - super! **Total**

Lunch - Healthy Eating Habits

L1. High-nutrient, low-carb lunch salads 5 times each week to fuel your body and curb cravings. Include:

1. Lean proteins (eggs, chicken, beef, fish, tofu, etc.) PLUS _____
2. Leafy greens (arugula, mixed greens) PLUS _____
3. Your favorite vinegarette dressing (apple, strawberry) _____
Optional: Low-sugar fruit (orange, berries, avocado, tomatoes) _____
Optional: Nuts / seeds _____
Optional - You drink low-sodium, low-carb soup (chick broth, miso soup) to help you feel fuller _____

Afternoon - Healthy Snacking Habits

A1. Drink 8 oz of water before snacking to curb cravings _____
A2. High-nutrient, low-calorie snacks – total calorie <300 _____
Optional If you drink non-water beverages, there's no added sugar (For coffee/tea, replace sugar/milk/cream with plant-based milk) _____
4 points - good start. 5-6 points - amazing!
7+ points - you are unstoppable in beating weight gain!   **Total** _____

Dinner - Healthy Eating Habits

D1. High-nutrient, low-carb dinner 5 times each week to fuel your body and curb cravings. Include:

1. Lean proteins (eggs, chicken, beef, fish, tofu, etc.) PLUS _____
2. Veggies rich in fiber, minerals, vitamins (green beans, spinach, celery, carrot, bok choy, etc.) _____
3. Minimally processed carbs (brown rice, whole grains) _____
Optional - Fresh fruit as desert _____
Bonus: No carbs or consume 50% less carbs than before _____
Bonus: Only use low-sodium salt / soy sauce for flavor _____
D2. No eating or snacking after 8pm your time _____
3 points - good start. 4-5 points - awesome! 6-7 points - excellent!   **Total** _____

Easy Calorie-Burning Habits
CB1. Worked out for 20-30 min and burned 200+ calories
You applied following techniques to prevent your metabolism from plateauing
a). Used more than 1 type of exercise machine   _____
b). Varied resistance and/or speed of the machine you used   _____
CB2. Instead of going to the gym, you did a 30-min brisk walk or 20-
min run or 20-min bike ride   _____
CB3. Did a 30-min sport   _____
CB4. Drank plenty of water after your exercise   _____
CB5. Walked at a moderate speed for 10+ min after lunch   _____
CB6. Took the stairs, skipped the elevator   _____
CB7. Walked at a moderate speed for 20+ min after dinner   _____
Bonus: Did 50 sit-ups and/or 20 push-ups (any style, lazy style) while
consuming digital content (e.g., listening to music, pod cast, watching
TV) at home   _____
Bonus: If you have an adjustable desk at home or work, you stood
while worked at your desk for 60+ minutes   _____
5 – 6 points - good start. 7 – 8 points – amazing!
9+ points - you are on fire!   **Total** _____

Night Time Healthy Habits and Sleep Hygiene
S1. Bedtime - No food past 3 hours & only drank water past 2 hours   _____
S2. Did a calming routine (e.g., meditation, warm bath, journaling,
stating affirmations, expressing gratitude, etc.)   _____
S3. Your bed area is device free (your cell phone, tablets, laptops are 5+
feet away and are all turned off)   _____
S4. Your room is noise free and dark once lights are off   _____
S5. Going to bed early to ensure at least 7 hours of sleep   _____
S6. Going to bed around the same time as previous days   _____
S7. Finished tracking points in each category today!   _____
4 points - good start. 5-6 points - great! 7+ points - excellent!   **Total** _____

Notes

Date: _____

Day 7

Give 1 point for each item and add total points for each category
Morning Ritual
Upon waking up, start your day with 1-minute positive mental conditioning exercises
MR1. Write down your affirmation in the present tense 3 times

_____

_____   _____

_____

MR2. Read your affirmation out loud in front a mirror and try to feel excited   _____
MR3. Express gratitude mentally or out loud 3 times. It can be as simple as "Thank you" or "I'm grateful for losing weight"   _____
1 point - good start. 2 points - awesome! 3 points excellent!   **Total**   _____

Morning - Healthy Eating Habits
M1. Before you eat or drink, record your weight here _____ lbs   _____

M2. Kickstart your metabolism, regulate your blood sugar, curb cravings - drink 8oz of warm water with
   a). Apple cider vinegar capsules OR
   b). Hand squeezed lemon juice   _____

M3. High-nutrient, low-carb breakfast. Include:
1. Lean protein (eggs, smoked salmon, plant based protein, etc.)   _____
2. Healthy fats (nuts, nut butter, seeds, avocado)   _____
3. Low-sugar raw fruit (orange, berries, melons, apple)   _____
4. Minimally processed carbs, high in fiber (whole grain/wheat)   _____
Optional: Low-sugar, low fat plant-based milk (almond)   _____
3-4 points - good start. 5-6 points - amazing! 7 points - super!   **Total**   _____

Lunch - Healthy Eating Habits

L1. High-nutrient, low-carb lunch salads 5 times each week to fuel your body and curb cravings. Include:

1. Lean proteins (eggs, chicken, beef, fish, tofu, etc.) PLUS _____

2. Leafy greens (arugula, mixed greens) PLUS _____

3. Your favorite vinegarette dressing (apple, strawberry) _____

Optional: Low-sugar fruit (orange, berries, avocado, tomatoes) _____

Optional: Nuts / seeds _____

Optional - You drink low-sodium, low-carb soup (chick broth, miso soup) to help you feel fuller _____

Afternoon - Healthy Snacking Habits

A1. Drink 8 oz of water before snacking to curb cravings _____

A2. High-nutrient, low-calorie snacks – total calorie <300 _____

Optional If you drink non-water beverages, there's no added sugar (For coffee/tea, replace sugar/milk/cream with plant-based milk) _____

4 points - good start. 5-6 points - amazing!

7+ points - you are unstoppable in beating weight gain!   **Total** _____

Dinner - Healthy Eating Habits

D1. High-nutrient, low-carb dinner 5 times each week to fuel your body and curb cravings. Include:

1. Lean proteins (eggs, chicken, beef, fish, tofu, etc.) PLUS _____

2. Veggies rich in fiber, minerals, vitamins (green beans, spinach, celery, carrot, bok choy, etc.) _____

3. Minimally processed carbs (brown rice, whole grains) _____

Optional - Fresh fruit as desert _____

Bonus: No carbs or consume 50% less carbs than before _____

Bonus: Only use low-sodium salt / soy sauce for flavor _____

D2. No eating or snacking after 8pm your time _____

3 points - good start. 4-5 points - awesome! 6-7 points - excellent!   **Total** _____

Easy Calorie-Burning Habits

CB1. Worked out for 20-30 min and burned 200+ calories
You applied following techniques to prevent your metabolism from plateauing
a). Used more than 1 type of exercise machine
b). Varied resistance and/or speed of the machine you used
CB2. Instead of going to the gym, you did a 30-min brisk walk or 20-min run or 20-min bike ride
CB3. Did a 30-min sport
CB4. Drank plenty of water after your exercise
CB5. Walked at a moderate speed for 10+ min after lunch
CB6. Took the stairs, skipped the elevator
CB7. Walked at a moderate speed for 20+ min after dinner
Bonus: Did 50 sit-ups and/or 20 push-ups (any style, lazy style) while consuming digital content (e.g., listening to music, pod cast, watching TV) at home
Bonus: If you have an adjustable desk at home or work, you stood while worked at your desk for 60+ minutes
5 – 6 points - good start. 7 – 8 points – amazing!
9+ points - you are on fire!   **Total**

Night Time Healthy Habits and Sleep Hygiene

S1. Bedtime - No food past 3 hours & only drank water past 2 hours
S2. Did a calming routine (e.g., meditation, warm bath, journaling, stating affirmations, expressing gratitude, etc.)
S3. Your bed area is device free (your cell phone, tablets, laptops are 5+ feet away and are all turned off)
S4. Your room is noise free and dark once lights are off
S5. Going to bed early to ensure at least 7 hours of sleep
S6. Going to bed around the same time as previous days
S7. Finished tracking points in each category today!
4 points - good start. 5-6 points - great! 7+ points - excellent!   **Total**

Notes

Date: _____

End of Week 3 Reflection

Day 1 weight _____   Day 7 weight _____

Which habit categories you ...	...consistently scored well?	...consistently scored lower (good start)?	...plan to improve the most next week?
Morning Ritual			
Morning Healthy Eating Habits			
Lunch Healthy Eating + Afternoon Healthy Snacking Habits			
Dinner Healthy Eating Habits			
Calorie-Burning Habits			
Night Time Healthy Habits and Sleep Hygiene			

Pat yourself on the back even if your weight roughly stayed the same this week. The fact that you have completed this entire week's habit tracking is a win! Celebrate every win, small or big. Just don't binge-eat your guilty pleasures. Take everything in moderation, and you will see and feel the rewards of a healthy lifestyle.

State these gratitude statements out loud 3 times and try to feel your weight loss outcomes and get excited:

- I am so grateful for being lighter, leaner, and more energetic!
- I am so grateful for completing daily habit tracking.
- I am so grateful for looking fabulous and feeling great.

149

Week 4

Date: _____

Day 1

Give 1 point for each item and add total points for each category
Morning Ritual
Upon waking up, start your day with 1-minute positive mental conditioning exercises
MR1. Write down your affirmation in the present tense 3 times

_____

_____

_____   _____

MR2. Read your affirmation out loud in front a mirror and try to feel excited   _____
MR3. Express gratitude mentally or out loud 3 times. It can be as simple as "Thank you" or "I'm grateful for losing weight"   _____
1 point - good start. 2 points - awesome! 3 points excellent!   **Total** _____

Morning - Healthy Eating Habits
M1. Before you eat or drink, record your weight here _____ lbs   _____

M2. Kickstart your metabolism, regulate your blood sugar, curb cravings - drink 8oz of warm water with
   a). Apple cider vinegar capsules OR
   b). Hand squeezed lemon juice   _____

M3. High-nutrient, low-carb breakfast. Include:

1. Lean protein (eggs, smoked salmon, plant based protein, etc)   _____
2. Healthy fats (nuts, nut butter, seeds, avocado)   _____
3. Low-sugar raw fruit (orange, berries, melons, apple)   _____
4. Minimally processed carbs, high in fiber (whole grain/wheat)   _____
Optional: Low-sugar, low fat plant-based milk (almond)   _____
3-4 points - good start. 5-6 points - amazing! 7 points - super!   **Total** _____

Lunch - Healthy Eating Habits

L1. High-nutrient, low-carb lunch salads 5 times each week to fuel your body and curb cravings. Include:

1. Lean proteins (eggs, chicken, beef, fish, tofu, etc.) PLUS _____

2. Leafy greens (arugula, mixed greens) PLUS _____

3. Your favorite vinegarette dressing (apple, strawberry) _____

Optional: Low-sugar fruit (orange, berries, avocado, tomatoes) _____

Optional: Nuts / seeds _____

Optional - You drink low-sodium, low-carb soup (chick broth, miso soup) to help you feel fuller _____

Afternoon - Healthy Snacking Habits

A1. Drink 8 oz of water before snacking to curb cravings _____

A2. High-nutrient, low-calorie snacks – total calorie <300 _____

Optional If you drink non-water beverages, there's no added sugar (For coffee/tea, replace sugar/milk/cream with plant-based milk) _____

4 points - good start. 5-6 points - amazing!

7+ points - you are unstoppable in beating weight gain! **Total** _____

Dinner - Healthy Eating Habits

D1. High-nutrient, low-carb dinner 5 times each week to fuel your body and curb cravings. Include:

1. Lean proteins (eggs, chicken, beef, fish, tofu, etc.) PLUS _____

2. Veggies rich in fiber, minerals, vitamins (green beans, spinach, celery, carrot, bok choy, etc.) _____

3. Minimally processed carbs (brown rice, whole grains) _____

Optional - Fresh fruit as desert _____

Bonus: No carbs or consume 50% less carbs than before _____

Bonus: Only use low-sodium salt / soy sauce for flavor _____

D2. No eating or snacking after 8pm your time _____

3 points - good start. 4-5 points - awesome! 6-7 points - excellent! **Total** _____

Easy Calorie-Burning Habits

CB1. Worked out for 20-30 min and burned 200+ calories

You applied following techniques to prevent your metabolism from plateauing

a). Used more than 1 type of exercise machine _____

b). Varied resistance and/or speed of the machine you used _____

CB2. Instead of going to the gym, you did a 30-min brisk walk or 20-min run or 20-min bike ride _____

CB3. Did a 30-min sport _____

CB4. Drank plenty of water after your exercise _____

CB5. Walked at a moderate speed for 10+ min after lunch _____

CB6. Took the stairs, skipped the elevator _____

CB7. Walked at a moderate speed for 20+ min after dinner _____

Bonus: Did 50 sit-ups and/or 20 push-ups (any style, lazy style) while consuming digital content (e.g., listening to music, pod cast, watching TV) at home _____

Bonus: If you have an adjustable desk at home or work, you stood while worked at your desk for 60+ minutes _____

5 – 6 points - good start. 7 – 8 points – amazing!

9+ points - you are on fire! **Total** _____

Night Time Healthy Habits and Sleep Hygiene

S1. Bedtime - No food past 3 hours & only drank water past 2 hours _____

S2. Did a calming routine (e.g., meditation, warm bath, journaling, stating affirmations, expressing gratitude, etc.) _____

S3. Your bed area is device free (your cell phone, tablets, laptops are 5+ feet away and are all turned off) _____

S4. Your room is noise free and dark once lights are off _____

S5. Going to bed early to ensure at least 7 hours of sleep _____

S6. Going to bed around the same time as previous days _____

S7. Finished tracking points in each category today! _____

4 points - good start. 5-6 points - great! 7+ points - excellent! **Total** _____

Notes

Date: _____

Day 2

Give 1 point for each item and add total points for each category

Morning Ritual

Upon waking up, start your day with 1-minute positive mental conditioning exercises

MR1. Write down your affirmation in the present tense 3 times

_____

_____

_____   _____

MR2. Read your affirmation out loud in front a mirror and try to feel excited   _____

MR3. Express gratitude mentally or out loud 3 times. It can be as simple as "Thank you" or "I'm grateful for losing weight"   _____

1 point - good start. 2 points - awesome! 3 points excellent!   **Total** ▬▬▬

Morning - Healthy Eating Habits

M1. Before you eat or drink, record your weight here _____ lbs   _____

M2. Kickstart your metabolism, regulate your blood sugar, curb cravings - drink 8oz of warm water with

   a). Apple cider vinegar capsules OR

   b). Hand squeezed lemon juice   _____

M3. High-nutrient, low-carb breakfast. Include:

1. Lean protein (eggs, smoked salmon, plant based protein, etc)   _____
2. Healthy fats (nuts, nut butter, seeds, avocado)   _____
3. Low-sugar raw fruit (orange, berries, melons, apple)   _____
4. Minimally processed carbs, high in fiber (whole grain/wheat)   _____

Optional: Low-sugar, low fat plant-based milk (almond)   _____

3-4 points - good start. 5-6 points - amazing! 7 points - super!   **Total** ▬▬▬

Lunch - Healthy Eating Habits

L1. High-nutrient, low-carb lunch salads 5 times each week to fuel your body and curb cravings. Include:

1. Lean proteins (eggs, chicken, beef, fish, tofu, etc.) PLUS   _____

2. Leafy greens (arugula, mixed greens) PLUS   _____

3. Your favorite vinegarette dressing (apple, strawberry)   _____

Optional: Low-sugar fruit (orange, berries, avocado, tomatoes)   _____

Optional: Nuts / seeds   _____

Optional - You drink low-sodium, low-carb soup (chick broth, miso soup) to help you feel fuller   _____

Afternoon - Healthy Snacking Habits

A1. Drink 8 oz of water before snacking to curb cravings   _____

A2. High-nutrient, low-calorie snacks – total calorie <300   _____

Optional If you drink non-water beverages, there's no added sugar (For coffee/tea, replace sugar/milk/cream with plant-based milk)   _____

4 points - good start. 5-6 points - amazing!

7+ points - you are unstoppable in beating weight gain!   **Total** _____

Dinner - Healthy Eating Habits

D1. High-nutrient, low-carb dinner 5 times each week to fuel your body and curb cravings. Include:

1. Lean proteins (eggs, chicken, beef, fish, tofu, etc.) PLUS   _____

2. Veggies rich in fiber, minerals, vitamins (green beans, spinach, celery, carrot, bok choy, etc.)   _____

3. Minimally processed carbs (brown rice, whole grains)   _____

Optional - Fresh fruit as desert   _____

Bonus: No carbs or consume 50% less carbs than before   _____

Bonus: Only use low-sodium salt / soy sauce for flavor   _____

D2. No eating or snacking after 8pm your time   _____

3 points - good start. 4-5 points - awesome! 6-7 points - excellent!   **Total** _____

Easy Calorie-Burning Habits
CB1. Worked out for 20-30 min and burned 200+ calories
You applied following techniques to prevent your metabolism from plateauing
a). Used more than 1 type of exercise machine _____
b). Varied resistance and/or speed of the machine you used _____
CB2. Instead of going to the gym, you did a 30-min brisk walk or 20-min run or 20-min bike ride
CB3. Did a 30-min sport _____
CB4. Drank plenty of water after your exercise _____
CB5. Walked at a moderate speed for 10+ min after lunch _____
CB6. Took the stairs, skipped the elevator _____
CB7. Walked at a moderate speed for 20+ min after dinner _____
Bonus: Did 50 sit-ups and/or 20 push-ups (any style, lazy style) while consuming digital content (e.g., listening to music, pod cast, watching TV) at home _____
Bonus: If you have an adjustable desk at home or work, you stood while worked at your desk for 60+ minutes _____
5 – 6 points - good start. 7 – 8 points – amazing!
9+ points - you are on fire! **Total** _____

Night Time Healthy Habits and Sleep Hygiene
S1. Bedtime - No food past 3 hours & only drank water past 2 hours _____
S2. Did a calming routine (e.g., meditation, warm bath, journaling, stating affirmations, expressing gratitude, etc.) _____
S3. Your bed area is device free (your cell phone, tablets, laptops are 5+ feet away and are all turned off) _____
S4. Your room is noise free and dark once lights are off _____
S5. Going to bed early to ensure at least 7 hours of sleep _____
S6. Going to bed around the same time as previous days _____
S7. Finished tracking points in each category today!
4 points - good start. 5-6 points - great! 7+ points - excellent! **Total** _____

Notes

_____

_____

_____

_____

_____

_____

_____

_____

Date: _____

Day 3

Give 1 point for each item and add total points for each category

Morning Ritual

Upon waking up, start your day with 1-minute positive mental conditioning exercises

MR1. Write down your affirmation in the present tense 3 times

_____

_____

_____   _____

MR2. Read your affirmation out loud in front a mirror and try to feel excited   _____

MR3. Express gratitude mentally or out loud 3 times. It can be as simple as "Thank you" or "I'm grateful for losing weight"   _____

1 point - good start. 2 points - awesome! 3 points excellent!   **Total**   _____

Morning - Healthy Eating Habits

M1. Before you eat or drink, record your weight here _____ lbs   _____

M2. Kickstart your metabolism, regulate your blood sugar, curb cravings - drink 8oz of warm water with

   a). Apple cider vinegar capsules OR

   b). Hand squeezed lemon juice   _____

M3. High-nutrient, low-carb breakfast. Include:

1. Lean protein (eggs, smoked salmon, plant-based protein, etc.)   _____
2. Healthy fats (nuts, nut butter, seeds, avocado)   _____
3. Low-sugar raw fruit (orange, berries, melons, apple)   _____
4. Minimally processed carbs, high in fiber (whole grain/wheat)   _____
Optional: Low-sugar, low fat plant-based milk (almond)   _____

3-4 points - good start. 5-6 points - amazing! 7 points - super!   **Total**   _____

Lunch - Healthy Eating Habits

L1. High-nutrient, low-carb lunch salads 5 times each week to fuel your body and curb cravings. Include:

1. Lean proteins (eggs, chicken, beef, fish, tofu, etc.) PLUS   _____

2. Leafy greens (arugula, mixed greens) PLUS   _____

3. Your favorite vinegarette dressing (apple, strawberry)   _____

Optional: Low-sugar fruit (orange, berries, avocado, tomatoes)   _____

Optional: Nuts / seeds   _____

Optional - You drink low-sodium, low-carb soup (chick broth, miso soup) to help you feel fuller   _____

Afternoon - Healthy Snacking Habits

A1. Drink 8 oz of water before snacking to curb cravings   _____

A2. High-nutrient, low-calorie snacks – total calorie <300   _____

Optional If you drink non-water beverages, there's no added sugar (For coffee/tea, replace sugar/milk/cream with plant-based milk)   _____

4 points - good start. 5-6 points - amazing!

7+ points - you are unstoppable in beating weight gain!   **Total** _____

Dinner - Healthy Eating Habits

D1. High-nutrient, low-carb dinner 5 times each week to fuel your body and curb cravings. Include:

1. Lean proteins (eggs, chicken, beef, fish, tofu, etc.) PLUS   _____

2. Veggies rich in fiber, minerals, vitamins (green beans, spinach, celery, carrot, bok choy, etc.)   _____

3. Minimally processed carbs (brown rice, whole grains)   _____

Optional - Fresh fruit as desert   _____

Bonus: No carbs or consume 50% less carbs than before   _____

Bonus: Only use low-sodium salt / soy sauce for flavor   _____

D2. No eating or snacking after 8pm your time   _____

3 points - good start. 4-5 points - awesome! 6-7 points - excellent!   **Total** _____

Easy Calorie-Burning Habits

CB1. Worked out for 20-30 min and burned 200+ calories
You applied following techniques to prevent your metabolism from plateauing
a). Used more than 1 type of exercise machine
b). Varied resistance and/or speed of the machine you used _____
CB2. Instead of going to the gym, you did a 30-min brisk walk or 20-min run or 20-min bike ride
CB3. Did a 30-min sport _____
CB4. Drank plenty of water after your exercise _____
CB5. Walked at a moderate speed for 10+ min after lunch _____
CB6. Took the stairs, skipped the elevator _____
CB7. Walked at a moderate speed for 20+ min after dinner _____
Bonus: Did 50 sit-ups and/or 20 push-ups (any style, lazy style) while consuming digital content (e.g., listening to music, pod cast, watching TV) at home _____
Bonus: If you have an adjustable desk at home or work, you stood while worked at your desk for 60+ minutes _____
5 – 6 points - good start. 7 – 8 points – amazing!
9+ points - you are on fire!   **Total** _____

Night Time Healthy Habits and Sleep Hygiene

S1. Bedtime - No food past 3 hours & only drank water past 2 hours _____
S2. Did a calming routine (e.g., meditation, warm bath, journaling, stating affirmations, expressing gratitude, etc.) _____
S3. Your bed area is device free (your cell phone, tablets, laptops are 5+ feet away and are all turned off)
S4. Your room is noise free and dark once lights are off _____
S5. Going to bed early to ensure at least 7 hours of sleep _____
S6. Going to bed around the same time as previous days _____
S7. Finished tracking points in each category today!
4 points - good start. 5-6 points - great! 7+ points - excellent!   **Total** _____

161

Notes

Date: _____

Day 4

Give 1 point for each item and add total points for each category

Morning Ritual

Upon waking up, start your day with 1-minute positive mental conditioning exercises

MR1. Write down your affirmation in the present tense 3 times

_____

_____

_____   _____

MR2. Read your affirmation out loud in front a mirror and try to feel excited   _____

MR3. Express gratitude mentally or out loud 3 times. It can be as simple as "Thank you" or "I'm grateful for losing weight"   _____

1 point - good start. 2 points - awesome! 3 points excellent!   **Total** _____

Morning - Healthy Eating Habits

M1. Before you eat or drink, record your weight here _____ lbs   _____

M2. Kickstart your metabolism, regulate your blood sugar, curb cravings - drink 8oz of warm water with

   a). Apple cider vinegar capsules OR

   b). Hand squeezed lemon juice   _____

M3. High-nutrient, low-carb breakfast. Include:

1. Lean protein (eggs, smoked salmon, plant-based protein, etc.)   _____
2. Healthy fats (nuts, nut butter, seeds, avocado)   _____
3. Low-sugar raw fruit (orange, berries, melons, apple)   _____
4. Minimally processed carbs, high in fiber (whole grain/wheat)   _____

Optional: Low-sugar, low fat plant-based milk (almond)   _____

3-4 points - good start. 5-6 points - amazing! 7 points - super!   **Total** _____

Lunch - Healthy Eating Habits

L1. High-nutrient, low-carb lunch salads 5 times each week to fuel your body and curb cravings. Include:

1. Lean proteins (eggs, chicken, beef, fish, tofu, etc.) PLUS   _____

2. Leafy greens (arugula, mixed greens) PLUS   _____

3. Your favorite vinegarette dressing (apple, strawberry)   _____

Optional: Low-sugar fruit (orange, berries, avocado, tomatoes)   _____

Optional: Nuts / seeds   _____

Optional - You drink low-sodium, low-carb soup (chick broth, miso soup) to help you feel fuller   _____

Afternoon - Healthy Snacking Habits

A1. Drink 8 oz of water before snacking to curb cravings   _____

A2. High-nutrient, low-calorie snacks – total calorie <300   _____

Optional If you drink non-water beverages, there's no added sugar (For coffee/tea, replace sugar/milk/cream with plant-based milk)   _____

4 points - good start. 5-6 points - amazing!

7+ points - you are unstoppable in beating weight gain!   **Total** _____

Dinner - Healthy Eating Habits

D1. High-nutrient, low-carb dinner 5 times each week to fuel your body and curb cravings. Include:

1. Lean proteins (eggs, chicken, beef, fish, tofu, etc.) PLUS   _____

2. Veggies rich in fiber, minerals, vitamins (green beans, spinach, celery, carrot, bok choy, etc.)   _____

3. Minimally processed carbs (brown rice, whole grains)   _____

Optional - Fresh fruit as desert   _____

Bonus: No carbs or consume 50% less carbs than before   _____

Bonus: Only use low-sodium salt / soy sauce for flavor   _____

D2. No eating or snacking after 8pm your time   _____

3 points - good start. 4-5 points - awesome! 6-7 points - excellent!   **Total** _____

Easy Calorie-Burning Habits

CB1. Worked out for 20-30 min and burned 200+ calories

You applied following techniques to prevent your metabolism from plateauing

a). Used more than 1 type of exercise machine _____

b). Varied resistance and/or speed of the machine you used _____

CB2. Instead of going to the gym, you did a 30-min brisk walk or 20-min run or 20-min bike ride _____

CB3. Did a 30-min sport _____

CB4. Drank plenty of water after your exercise _____

CB5. Walked at a moderate speed for 10+ min after lunch _____

CB6. Took the stairs, skipped the elevator _____

CB7. Walked at a moderate speed for 20+ min after dinner _____

Bonus: Did 50 sit-ups and/or 20 push-ups (any style, lazy style) while consuming digital content (e.g., listening to music, pod cast, watching TV) at home _____

Bonus: If you have an adjustable desk at home or work, you stood while worked at your desk for 60+ minutes _____

5 – 6 points - good start. 7 – 8 points – amazing!

9+ points - you are on fire! **Total** _____

Night Time Healthy Habits and Sleep Hygiene

S1. Bedtime - No food past 3 hours & only drank water past 2 hours _____

S2. Did a calming routine (e.g., meditation, warm bath, journaling, stating affirmations, expressing gratitude, etc.) _____

S3. Your bed area is device free (your cell phone, tablets, laptops are 5+ feet away and are all turned off) _____

S4. Your room is noise free and dark once lights are off _____

S5. Going to bed early to ensure at least 7 hours of sleep _____

S6. Going to bed around the same time as previous days _____

S7. Finished tracking points in each category today! _____

4 points - good start. 5-6 points - great! 7+ points - excellent! **Total** _____

Notes

Date: _____

Day 5

Give 1 point for each item and add total points for each category

Morning Ritual

Upon waking up, start your day with 1-minute positive mental conditioning exercises

MR1. Write down your affirmation in the present tense 3 times

_____

_____

_____   _____

MR2. Read your affirmation out loud in front a mirror and try to feel excited

MR3. Express gratitude mentally or out loud 3 times. It can be as simple as "Thank you" or "I'm grateful for losing weight"

1 point - good start. 2 points - awesome! 3 points excellent!   **Total**   ▬▬▬

Morning - Healthy Eating Habits

M1. Before you eat or drink, record your weight here _____ lbs   _____

M2. Kickstart your metabolism, regulate your blood sugar, curb cravings - drink 8oz of warm water with

   a). Apple cider vinegar capsules OR

   b). Hand squeezed lemon juice   _____

M3. High-nutrient, low-carb breakfast. Include:

1. Lean protein (eggs, smoked salmon, plant based protein, etc.)   _____
2. Healthy fats (nuts, nut butter, seeds, avocado)   _____
3. Low-sugar raw fruit (orange, berries, melons, apple)   _____
4. Minimally processed carbs, high in fiber (whole grain/wheat)   _____

Optional: Low-sugar, low fat plant-based milk (almond)   _____

3-4 points - good start. 5-6 points - amazing! 7 points - super!   **Total**   ▬▬▬

Lunch - Healthy Eating Habits

L1. High-nutrient, low-carb lunch salads 5 times each week to fuel your body and curb cravings. Include:

1. Lean proteins (eggs, chicken, beef, fish, tofu, etc.) PLUS ⎯⎯⎯⎯⎯

2. Leafy greens (arugula, mixed greens) PLUS ⎯⎯⎯⎯⎯

3. Your favorite vinegarette dressing (apple, strawberry) ⎯⎯⎯⎯⎯

Optional: Low-sugar fruit (orange, berries, avocado, tomatoes) ⎯⎯⎯⎯⎯

Optional: Nuts / seeds ⎯⎯⎯⎯⎯

Optional - You drink low-sodium, low-carb soup (chick broth, miso soup) to help you feel fuller ⎯⎯⎯⎯⎯

Afternoon - Healthy Snacking Habits

A1. Drink 8 oz of water before snacking to curb cravings ⎯⎯⎯⎯⎯

A2. High-nutrient, low-calorie snacks – total calorie <300 ⎯⎯⎯⎯⎯

Optional If you drink non-water beverages, there's no added sugar (For coffee/tea, replace sugar/milk/cream with plant-based milk) ⎯⎯⎯⎯⎯

4 points - good start. 5-6 points - amazing!

7+ points - you are unstoppable in beating weight gain!   **Total** ⎯⎯⎯⎯⎯

Dinner - Healthy Eating Habits

D1. High-nutrient, low-carb dinner 5 times each week to fuel your body and curb cravings. Include:

1. Lean proteins (eggs, chicken, beef, fish, tofu, etc.) PLUS ⎯⎯⎯⎯⎯

2. Veggies rich in fiber, minerals, vitamins (green beans, spinach, celery, carrot, bok choy, etc.) ⎯⎯⎯⎯⎯

3. Minimally processed carbs (brown rice, whole grains) ⎯⎯⎯⎯⎯

Optional - Fresh fruit as desert ⎯⎯⎯⎯⎯

Bonus: No carbs or consume 50% less carbs than before ⎯⎯⎯⎯⎯

Bonus: Only use low-sodium salt / soy sauce for flavor ⎯⎯⎯⎯⎯

D2. No eating or snacking after 8pm your time ⎯⎯⎯⎯⎯

3 points - good start. 4-5 points - awesome! 6-7 points - excellent!   **Total** ⎯⎯⎯⎯⎯

Easy Calorie-Burning Habits

CB1. Worked out for 20-30 min and burned 200+ calories
You applied following techniques to prevent your metabolism from plateauing
a). Used more than 1 type of exercise machine
b). Varied resistance and/or speed of the machine you used _____
CB2. Instead of going to the gym, you did a 30-min brisk walk or 20-min run or 20-min bike ride
CB3. Did a 30-min sport _____
CB4. Drank plenty of water after your exercise _____
CB5. Walked at a moderate speed for 10+ min after lunch
CB6. Took the stairs, skipped the elevator _____
CB7. Walked at a moderate speed for 20+ min after dinner _____
Bonus: Did 50 sit-ups and/or 20 push-ups (any style, lazy style) while consuming digital content (e.g., listening to music, pod cast, watching TV) at home _____
Bonus: If you have an adjustable desk at home or work, you stood while worked at your desk for 60+ minutes _____
5 – 6 points - good start. 7 – 8 points – amazing!
9+ points - you are on fire!   **Total** _____

Night Time Healthy Habits and Sleep Hygiene

S1. Bedtime - No food past 3 hours & only drank water past 2 hours _____
S2. Did a calming routine (e.g., meditation, warm bath, journaling, stating affirmations, expressing gratitude, etc.) _____
S3. Your bed area is device free (your cell phone, tablets, laptops are 5+ feet away and are all turned off) _____
S4. Your room is noise free and dark once lights are off _____
S5. Going to bed early to ensure at least 7 hours of sleep _____
S6. Going to bed around the same time as previous days _____
S7. Finished tracking points in each category today! _____
4 points - good start. 5-6 points - great! 7+ points - excellent!   **Total** _____

Notes

Date: _____

Day 6

Give 1 point for each item and add total points for each category

Morning Ritual

Upon waking up, start your day with 1-minute positive mental conditioning exercises

MR1. Write down your affirmation in the present tense 3 times

_____

_____

_____   _____

MR2. Read your affirmation out loud in front a mirror and try to feel excited   _____

MR3. Express gratitude mentally or out loud 3 times. It can be as simple as "Thank you" or "I'm grateful for losing weight"   _____

1 point - good start. 2 points - awesome! 3 points excellent!   **Total** _____

Morning - Healthy Eating Habits

M1. Before you eat or drink, record your weight here _____ lbs   _____

M2. Kickstart your metabolism, regulate your blood sugar, curb cravings - drink 8oz of warm water with

  a). Apple cider vinegar capsules OR

  b). Hand squeezed lemon juice   _____

M3. High-nutrient, low-carb breakfast. Include:

1. Lean protein (eggs, smoked salmon, plant-based protein, etc.)   _____
2. Healthy fats (nuts, nut butter, seeds, avocado)   _____
3. Low-sugar raw fruit (orange, berries, melons, apple)   _____
4. Minimally processed carbs, high in fiber (whole grain/wheat)   _____
Optional: Low-sugar, low fat plant-based milk (almond)   _____
3-4 points - good start. 5-6 points - amazing! 7 points - super!   **Total** _____

Lunch - Healthy Eating Habits

L1. High-nutrient, low-carb lunch salads 5 times each week to fuel your body and curb cravings. Include:

1. Lean proteins (eggs, chicken, beef, fish, tofu, etc.) PLUS   _____

2. Leafy greens (arugula, mixed greens) PLUS   _____

3. Your favorite vinegarette dressing (apple, strawberry)   _____

Optional: Low-sugar fruit (orange, berries, avocado, tomatoes)   _____

Optional: Nuts / seeds   _____

Optional - You drink low-sodium, low-carb soup (chick broth, miso soup) to help you feel fuller   _____

Afternoon - Healthy Snacking Habits

A1. Drink 8 oz of water before snacking to curb cravings   _____

A2. High-nutrient, low-calorie snacks – total calorie <300   _____

Optional If you drink non-water beverages, there's no added sugar (For coffee/tea, replace sugar/milk/cream with plant-based milk)   _____

4 points - good start. 5-6 points - amazing!

7+ points - you are unstoppable in beating weight gain!   **Total** _____

Dinner - Healthy Eating Habits

D1. High-nutrient, low-carb dinner 5 times each week to fuel your body and curb cravings. Include:

1. Lean proteins (eggs, chicken, beef, fish, tofu, etc.) PLUS   _____

2. Veggies rich in fiber, minerals, vitamins (green beans, spinach, celery, carrot, bok choy, etc.)   _____

3. Minimally processed carbs (brown rice, whole grains)   _____

Optional - Fresh fruit as desert   _____

Bonus: No carbs or consume 50% less carbs than before   _____

Bonus: Only use low-sodium salt / soy sauce for flavor   _____

D2. No eating or snacking after 8pm your time   _____

3 points - good start. 4-5 points - awesome! 6-7 points - excellent!   **Total** _____

Easy Calorie-Burning Habits

CB1. Worked out for 20-30 min and burned 200+ calories
You applied following techniques to prevent your metabolism from plateauing
a). Used more than 1 type of exercise machine _____
b). Varied resistance and/or speed of the machine you used _____
CB2. Instead of going to the gym, you did a 30-min brisk walk or 20-min run or 20-min bike ride _____
CB3. Did a 30-min sport _____
CB4. Drank plenty of water after your exercise _____
CB5. Walked at a moderate speed for 10+ min after lunch _____
CB6. Took the stairs, skipped the elevator _____
CB7. Walked at a moderate speed for 20+ min after dinner _____
Bonus: Did 50 sit-ups and/or 20 push-ups (any style, lazy style) while consuming digital content (e.g., listening to music, pod cast, watching TV) at home _____
Bonus: If you have an adjustable desk at home or work, you stood while worked at your desk for 60+ minutes _____
5 – 6 points - good start. 7 – 8 points – amazing!
9+ points - you are on fire! **Total** _____

Night Time Healthy Habits and Sleep Hygiene

S1. Bedtime - No food past 3 hours & only drank water past 2 hours _____
S2. Did a calming routine (e.g., meditation, warm bath, journaling, stating affirmations, expressing gratitude, etc.) _____
S3. Your bed area is device free (your cell phone, tablets, laptops are 5+ feet away and are all turned off) _____
S4. Your room is noise free and dark once lights are off _____
S5. Going to bed early to ensure at least 7 hours of sleep _____
S6. Going to bed around the same time as previous days _____
S7. Finished tracking points in each category today! _____
4 points - good start. 5-6 points - great! 7+ points - excellent! **Total** _____

Notes

Date: _____

Day 7

Give 1 point for each item and add total points for each category

Morning Ritual

Upon waking up, start your day with 1-minute positive mental conditioning exercises

MR1. Write down your affirmation in the present tense 3 times

_____

_____

_____   _____

MR2. Read your affirmation out loud in front a mirror and try to feel excited   _____

MR3. Express gratitude mentally or out loud 3 times. It can be as simple as "Thank you" or "I'm grateful for losing weight"   _____

1 point - good start. 2 points - awesome! 3 points excellent!   **Total**   _____

Morning - Healthy Eating Habits

M1. Before you eat or drink, record your weight here _____ lbs   _____

M2. Kickstart your metabolism, regulate your blood sugar, curb cravings - drink 8oz of warm water with

   a). Apple cider vinegar capsules OR

   b). Hand squeezed lemon juice   _____

M3. High-nutrient, low-carb breakfast. Include:

1. Lean protein (eggs, smoked salmon, plant based protein, etc.)   _____
2. Healthy fats (nuts, nut butter, seeds, avocado)   _____
3. Low-sugar raw fruit (orange, berries, melons, apple)   _____
4. Minimally processed carbs, high in fiber (whole grain/wheat)   _____

Optional: Low-sugar, low fat plant-based milk (almond)   _____

3-4 points - good start. 5-6 points - amazing! 7 points - super!   **Total**   _____

Lunch - Healthy Eating Habits

L1. High-nutrient, low-carb lunch salads 5 times each week to fuel your body and curb cravings. Include:

1. Lean proteins (eggs, chicken, beef, fish, tofu, etc.) PLUS _____

2. Leafy greens (arugula, mixed greens) PLUS _____

3. Your favorite vinegarette dressing (apple, strawberry) _____

Optional: Low-sugar fruit (orange, berries, avocado, tomatoes) _____

Optional: Nuts / seeds _____

Optional - You drink low-sodium, low-carb soup (chick broth, miso soup) to help you feel fuller _____

Afternoon - Healthy Snacking Habits

A1. Drink 8 oz of water before snacking to curb cravings _____

A2. High-nutrient, low-calorie snacks – total calorie <300 _____

Optional If you drink non-water beverages, there's no added sugar (For coffee/tea, replace sugar/milk/cream with plant-based milk) _____

4 points - good start. 5-6 points - amazing!

7+ points - you are unstoppable in beating weight gain! **Total** _____

Dinner - Healthy Eating Habits

D1. High-nutrient, low-carb dinner 5 times each week to fuel your body and curb cravings. Include:

1. Lean proteins (eggs, chicken, beef, fish, tofu, etc.) PLUS _____

2. Veggies rich in fiber, minerals, vitamins (green beans, spinach, celery, carrot, bok choy, etc.) _____

3. Minimally processed carbs (brown rice, whole grains) _____

Optional - Fresh fruit as desert _____

Bonus: No carbs or consume 50% less carbs than before _____

Bonus: Only use low-sodium salt / soy sauce for flavor _____

D2. No eating or snacking after 8pm your time _____

3 points - good start. 4-5 points - awesome! 6-7 points - excellent! **Total** _____

Easy Calorie-Burning Habits

CB1. Worked out for 20-30 min and burned 200+ calories

You applied following techniques to prevent your metabolism from plateauing

a). Used more than 1 type of exercise machine _____

b). Varied resistance and/or speed of the machine you used _____

CB2. Instead of going to the gym, you did a 30-min brisk walk or 20-min run or 20-min bike ride _____

CB3. Did a 30-min sport _____

CB4. Drank plenty of water after your exercise _____

CB5. Walked at a moderate speed for 10+ min after lunch _____

CB6. Took the stairs, skipped the elevator _____

CB7. Walked at a moderate speed for 20+ min after dinner _____

Bonus: Did 50 sit-ups and/or 20 push-ups (any style, lazy style) while consuming digital content (e.g., listening to music, pod cast, watching TV) at home _____

Bonus: If you have an adjustable desk at home or work, you stood while worked at your desk for 60+ minutes _____

5 – 6 points - good start. 7 – 8 points – amazing!

9+ points - you are on fire!   **Total** _____

Night Time Healthy Habits and Sleep Hygiene

S1. Bedtime - No food past 3 hours & only drank water past 2 hours _____

S2. Did a calming routine (e.g., meditation, warm bath, journaling, stating affirmations, expressing gratitude, etc.) _____

S3. Your bed area is device free (your cell phone, tablets, laptops are 5+ feet away and are all turned off) _____

S4. Your room is noise free and dark once lights are off _____

S5. Going to bed early to ensure at least 7 hours of sleep _____

S6. Going to bed around the same time as previous days _____

S7. Finished tracking points in each category today! _____

4 points - good start. 5-6 points - great! 7+ points - excellent!   **Total** _____

Notes

Date: _____

End of Week 4 Reflection

Day 1 weight _____   Day 7 weight _____

Which habit categories you ...	...consistently scored well?	...consistently scored lower (good start)?	...plan to improve the most next week?
Morning Ritual			
Morning Healthy Eating Habits			
Lunch Healthy Eating + Afternoon Healthy Snacking Habits			
Dinner Healthy Eating Habits			
Calorie-Burning Habits			
Night Time Healthy Habits and Sleep Hygiene			

Regardless of weight change, the fact that you have completed this entire week's habit tracking is a win! Pat yourself on the back for completing this 28-day journey. Celebrate every win, small or big. Just don't binge-eat your guilty pleasures. Take everything in moderation, and you will see and feel the rewards of living a healthy lifestyle.

State these gratitude statements out loud 3 times and try to feel your weight loss outcomes and get excited:

- I am so grateful for feeling lighter, leaner, and more energetic!
- I am so grateful for putting high-nutrient foods in my body and keeping myself active.
- I am so grateful for living this healthy lifestyle.

Conclusion

Congratulations on embarking on this 28-day weight loss journey! Regardless of how many pounds you have lost or will lose by following the instructions in this journal, I am so excited for you. This journal is more than a tool; it is also a turning point in your life. Here, you're not just aiming to end the weight loss saga but setting the stage for lasting health and vitality. I trust you will reach your desired weight. If you ever feel tempted to return to your old habits, please revisit this journal, your secret weapon, to resume healthier living.

After you finish writing in this journal and you would like to start a new 28-day cycle of journaling, planning, and tracking, you can get the standalone *Weight Loss Hacks for Women Journal* in the paperback format by scanning the QR code below.

Your Voice Matters!

If you find value in this book and its approach to weight loss, I'd appreciate you sharing your feedback with a review of this journal. Your feedback not only assists others in discovering easy and sustainable solutions but also contributes to a community of positivity and support.

Your positive reflections can inspire positive changes in others and attract more positivity to your life. Leaving your rating/review on this book is quick and easy. Please leave your rating/review now.

Thank you!

- Your weight loss partner and biggest cheerleader, Kate M. Right.

P.S. If you're interested in exploring additional insights and hacks for your physical, mental, and emotional well-being, I invite you to join a community of like-minded individuals at harmonybookpub.com.

At harmonybookpub.com, you'll find a curated collection of my writings and upcoming books designed to enlighten you and enhance your journey of personal transformation.

Made in the USA
Middletown, DE
03 December 2024

66029423R00109